Contents

Introduction

Chapter 1. Underlying Causes of Parkinson's   15

The Brain   15
Free Radicals and Anti-Oxidants   16
Anti-oxidants   18
Genetics   19
Parkinson's and Inheritance Factors   20
Young-onset Parkinson's Disease   20
Other Factors   21
Low Levels of Estrogen   21
Caffeine and Nicotine   22
Diet and Nutrition   22
Age Related Factors   23

Chapter 2. The Diagnosis of Parkinson's Disease   25

The main characteristics of Parkinson's   25
Tremor   25
Rigidity   26
Bradykinesia   26
Balance   27
The process of elimination   27
Carrying Out the Diagnosis   28
Assessing the Symptom   28
Consider all the Possible Diagnosis   28

Chapter 3. Medication   31

Medications   31

Drugs that Replace Dopamine   32
Enzyme Inhibitors   32
Dopamine Agents   33
Anticholinergic Drugs   33
Amantadine   34
Using medications safely   34

Chapter 4. Surgery and Ongoing Research   37

Surgery and Parkinson's Disease   37
Deep Brain Stimulation   37
Lesioning-Pallidotomy and Thalamotomy   38
Cell Implants   38
Stem Cells from Embryos   39
Growth Factors   40

Chapter 5. Finding the Right GP/Consultant   41

Chapter 6. Combating Depression   45

Parkinson's and Depression   45
Factors Contributing to Depression   45
The Importance of Working Towards   46
Acceptance of Parkinson's
The Importance of Support Groups   47

Chapter 7. Diet and Parkinson's Disease   53

Eating Well With Parkinson's   53
Underweight   55
Dishes and Cutlery   56
Advice on Eating and Swallowing Food   57
Tips on Easy Swallowing   57
Puree Diets   58
A Sample Eating Plan   59

T   L

Emerald Publishing
Brighton BN7 2SH

ISBN 9781847162199

Printed by GN Digital Books Essex

Cover design by Bookworks Islington

Parkinson's Medication and the Interaction with Food   60
Controlling Nausea   60
Vitamins and Minerals   61

Chapter 8. Exercise and Parkinson's   63

The Benefits of exercise and Parkinson's   63
Putting Together an Exercise Plan   63
Aerobic Fitness   64
Improving Muscle Strength   65
Flexibility   66
Starting Your Exercises   67

Chapter 9. Welfare Benefits and Employment   69

Disability Living Allowance   69
The Care Component   70
The Mobility Component   70
Claiming the Allowance   70
Attendance Allowance   71
Claiming Attendance Allowance   71
Benefits Payable if You Cannot Work Because of
Illness Disability, Age or Caring Responsibilities   72
Statutory Sick Pay   72
How Average Earnings Are Worked Out   72
Salary Sacrifice Scheme and SSP   73
Agency Workers   73
Statutory Sick pay rates   74
Employment and Support Allowance   74
Rates of ESA   75
Customers Moving onto ESA from Incapacity Benefits   76
Pension Income Rules   76
Income Tax   77
State Pension   77
NI Contributions Towards a Basic State Pension   79

NI Contributions that Do Not Count   80
Class 1 Contributions   80
Class 2 Contributions   81
NI Contribution Credits   81
Class 3 Contributions   82
National Insurance Credits   82
The State Pension Age   84
State Pensions for People over 80   86
Additional State Pension   86
Contracting Out   87
Increasing Your State Pension   88
Filling Gaps in Your Record   88
Deferring Your State Pension   89
Carers Allowance   90
Top Up Benefits   90
Income Support   91
Income Support Rates   91
Further Premiums   92
Pension Credits   92
Housing Benefits   93
Changes to Housing Benefits After April 2011   95
Council Tax   96
Working Tax Credit   97
Job-Seekers Allowance   98
Other Benefits Available   99
The Social Fund   99
Winter Fuel Payments   100

Chapter 10. Living and Coping With Parkinson's   101

General Advice   101
Therapies for Parkinson's Disease   102
Physiotherapy   102
Occupational Therapy   103
Speech and Language Therapists   104

Driving and Parkinson's   104
Parkinson's Medication and Driving   105
Mobility Centres and Driving Assessment   105
Priority parking and The Blue Badge Scheme   106
Car Insurance and Parkinson's   106
Adaptations to Vehicles for people With Parkinson's   107
Dropped Kerbs   107
Employment and Parkinson's   108
The Equality Act 2010   108

Chapter 11. People Who Care for Parkinson's Sufferers   109

Definition of a Carer   109
Providing Care to a Person With Parkinson's   109
Talking to Health Professionals   110
The Carers Register   111
Time Off From Caring   111
Carers Assessment   112
Carers and Employment Rights   112
Telling Your Employer About Your Role as a Carer   112
Statutory Rights for Carers   113
Websites for Carers   114

Useful Addresses

Appendix one.
Medication Logs

Index

Explaining Parkinson's
Introduction

A good deal has been written about Parkinson's over the years, and there are many avenues through which information about the condition can be obtained. Throughout this book, I will be referring to various organisations that play a major role in providing invaluable information about Parkinson's disease.

My own background is non-medical so it should be understood from the outset that what you read in this book is in no way based on medical opinion, it is just a product of research and personal experiences. My personal experiences have involved my partner's relatives and very close friends of mine and I have been deeply involved in all aspects of Parkinson's from initial diagnosis to living with Parkinson's and medication and ongoing needs and support.

In addition to this, I myself was diagnosed mistakenly with Parkinson's disease by my doctor (although I hasten to add this was an initial diagnosis and he referred me to a specialist who, after a few months of tests, and a deep brain scan, informed me that I did not in fact have Parkinson's). What this little episode did was take me through the initial phase of trauma and then acceptance that I might have Parkinson's disease. It was the culmination of all these experiences that prompted me, with the aid of my partner, to write this book.

What is Parkinson's?

Parkinson's is (one of) the most common disorders of the nervous system. Muscle movements are affected with the main symptoms being tremors, stiffening of the muscles and, overall, slower movement patterns. Parkinson's was first identified in 1817 by Doctor James Parkinson, working in London. Although the condition has been in existence for a very long time, it is now more prevalent because of the aging population, the fact that people are living longer. It is recognised most frequently in people of 60 or over, although it is also prevalent in some younger people.

Doctors are now far more aware of Parkinson's and the advances in drugs available to treat them have been very significant, particularly in the last decade. Research nowadays is focussed on slowing and preventing the progression of the condition and there will be corresponding advances in the types of medication available.

This brief book covers the diagnosis of Parkinson's, dealing with the condition in its early stages and explaining the condition to others, choosing the most effective medication for you, choosing diet and putting together an exercise regime, a discussion of surgical options and also the financial aspects of Parkinson's such as benefits and employment. There is a section about people who care for those with Parkinson's and many useful contacts.

Initially, a lot of medical terminology is used and I do my best to elaborate on the meanings of various terms. I sincerely hope that you will benefit from this brief but nonetheless important and informative book .

Doreen Jarrett 2011

Chapter 1

The Underlying Causes of Parkinson's

As was mentioned in the introduction, Parkinson's was identified almost 200 years ago. However, as with a lot of illnesses, the exact cause of the condition remains a mystery, notwithstanding lots of research, and a number of factors are seen as contributory.

The brain

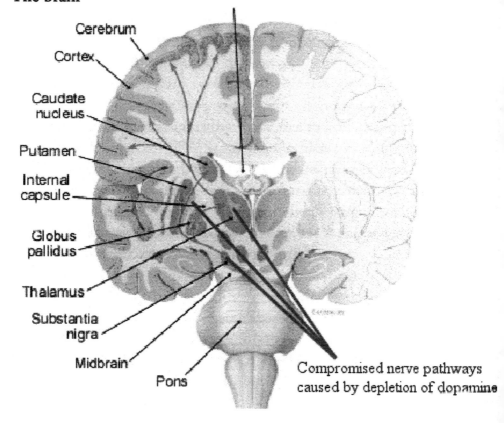

Cerebrum

Cortex

Caudate nucleus

Putamen

Internal capsule

Globus pallidus

Thalamus

Substantia nigra

Midbrain

Pons

Compromised nerve pathways caused by depletion of dopamine

The root of Parkinson's lies within the brain. Obviously, it is very difficult to treat the brain in a mechanistic way as it incorporates our mind and is our very existence. However, scientific research has determined that bodily movements are regulated by an area of the brain called the basal ganglia, whose cells require a proper balance of substances known as *dopamine* and *acetylcholine*, both involved in the transmission of nerve impulses. With Parkinson's, cells that produce dopamine begin to degenerate. When this happens, the insufficient dopamine disturbs the balance between dopamine and other transmitters, such as acetylcholine.

Therefore, dopamine can be seen as a chemical messenger responsible for transmitting signals between the substantia nigra and the next 'relay station' of the brain, which is the corpus striatum, to produce smooth, purposeful muscle activity. Loss of dopamine causes the nerve cells of the striatum to fire out of control, leaving the person unable to direct or control their movements in a normal manner.

The exact cause of this cell death or impairment is unknown. However, scientists have made advances in this area and one theory holds that free radicals, unstable and potentially damaging molecules generated by normal chemical reactions in the body, may contribute to nerve cell death that leads to Parkinson's.

Free Radicals and Anti-Oxidants

Free radicals are the highly unstable chemicals that attack, infiltrate and ultimately injure vital cell structures. Most stable chemical compounds in the body possess a pair of electrons.

Sometimes, one member of the electron pair gets stripped away. The resulting compound (less one electron) is called a free radical.

The term 'free radical' means that it is now free to combine with another element to form a new stable compound. Free radicals can do a lot of damage by forming a chain reaction and breaking down other cell structures. A good comparison is that of the family unit. When two people join together and form a family unit, they are not usually available to other partners. However, if they separate the partners can go and look for another mate. Potentially, they can break up another stable marriage. This is the way free radicals work. When a free radical is born, it goes around the body looking for another compound to steal an electron from. While on the prowl, these free radicals can do tremendous damage to cells.

The most observed free radical chain reaction in living things is lipid peroxidation. The term lipid refers to any fat-soluble substance, animal or vegetable. Peroxidation means the formation of a peroxide molecule. These are the molecules with the greatest proportion of oxygen molecules.

Ninety-eight percent of the oxygen we breathe is used by tiny powerhouses within our cells called mitochondria, that convert sugar, fats and inorganic phosphate oxygen into adenosine triphosphate the universal form of energy that we need to live. This energy producing activity of the mitochondria involves a series of intricate complex and vital biochemical processes dependent on vast numbers of enzymes. These in turn are dependent upon dozens of nutrient factors and co-factors. In this metabolism process a very small amount of left over oxygen loses electrons, creating free radicals. These free radicals burn holes in our cellular membranes. Calcium penetrates our cells through these holes. This excess calcium results in cell death. This in turn weakens tissues and organs with the body, in turn weakening our overall immunity and resistance.

In addition to the oxygen that we breathe, the free radicals can also come from such things as environmental pollution, radiation, cigarette smoke, chemicals and herbicides.

Fundamental to having a healthy body is repairing the damage caused by the free radicals before it is too late and to protect the body's tissue cells from the free radicals before they cause mutations.

Antioxidants

Antioxidants are substances that have free radical chain reaction breaking properties. The antioxidants deactivate potentially dangerous free radicals before they can damage cells machinery. Most of these antioxidants come from plants and are called Phytochemicals. Among the most effective are vitamin A, C and E (known as the ACE trio against cancer). Out of these, vitamin C is the most effective.

Each cell produces its own antioxidants. However, the ability to produce them decreases with age. That is why (see the chapter on diet) a diet rich in antioxidant and phytochemical rich fruits and vegetables supplemented with additional vitamins and minerals is important.

Genetics

Researchers think, as do a lot of doctor's, that Parkinson's has a genetic link. The genetic material that makes us who and what we are is stored in our chromosomes. Chromosomes consist of deoxyribonucleic acid (DNA) which in turn consists of genes, which are the blueprints for our inherited traits such as the colour of our eyes, height and numerous other characteristics and conditions such as cancers and diabetes. A number of studies have taken place to try to determine the genetic link but most have been inconclusive.

When assessing whether a disease is inherited, researchers will examine family history. It appears that the genetic link is strongest with first-degree relatives, i.e. parents, siblings and children. The larger the number of relatives with a specific condition the greater the likelihood that a genetic factor has played a direct role in transmission.

When it comes to Parkinson's, however, it seems that the jury is out and that there are differing opinions as to the importance of the genetic link. Some families have a clear pattern of Parkinson's disease within the family tree. Multiple family members across the generations have the condition.

A study of a family, the Contursi family, revealed that 60 family members had Parkinson's disease over five generations. Autopsies of several family members showed the classic loss of dopamine cells and the presence of Lewy bodies.

Parkinson's disease and inheritance factors

The chart below, compiled by Dr Jill Marjama-Lyons clearly demonstrates the risks of inheriting Parkinson's disease based on family history.

Person with Parkinson's disease in your family	Chance of getting Parkinson's disease
None	1-2 per cent, same as the general population
Brother or sister	5-6 per cent
One parent	10 per cent
Parent and sibling	20-40 per cent

As the table demonstrates, even if some family members have Parkinson's disease, there is no reason to assume that other family members will develop it as well. The risk may increase but there is nothing concrete by way of research to prove that this is absolutely the case.

Young-onset Parkinson's disease

Parkinson's disease is not solely a disease of the elderly. While the majority of cases are diagnosed in older people, it is estimated that about 15 per cent of people with Parkinson's disease develop symptoms before the age of 50. It has been established that the rate of young-onset Parkinson's disease is on the rise. Those who develop the disease prior to 55 years of age are considered to have young-onset Parkinson's disease. Very rarely, people under 21 will develop the disease, which is then classified as juvenile-onset Parkinson's disease.

Other factors

Research has been carried out on the influence of the environment as a factor in contributing to Parkinson's disease. There is no clear evidence to suggest that environment is major factor. Relatively weak influences have shown to be a possible factor, such as drinking water from a well, the proximity to wood mills, and the associated chemicals employed in these mills and also exposure to herbicides and pesticides, particularly among agricultural workers. However, such factors only contribute to a very small minority of cases.

Exposure to heavy metals, occupational exposure, such as copper, lead, iron, manganese and so on, increases the risk of developing Parkinson's by up to 10 times compared to the normal population. In addition, the iron and aluminium content is much higher than normal in the brains of people with Parkinson's disease.

Viral infections may also play a role in triggering Parkinson's disease. For example, during the outbreak of sleeping sickness during the First World War, about 15 million people were infected with the virus, and about 6 million of those developed Parkinson's symptoms. However, it was found later, during autopsies of some of the victims that the symptoms, although similar, weren't in fact Parkinson's.

Low levels of Estrogen

Some researchers believe that the female hormone estrogen may help protect against developing Parkinson's disease. This connection was supported by research published in the American journal *Movement Disorders* which compared the medical records of 72 women with Parkinson's disease and a group of women the same age who did not have the disease. The researchers found that the women who developed Parkinson's had three times the rate of hysterectomies, a higher rate of early menopause, and a lower rate of estrogen replacement therapy after menopause. The study suggested that estrogen may help to prevent or delay the onset of Parkinson's disease.

Caffeine and nicotine

Caffeine has been blamed for many negative health effects. However, it has also been associated with a lower rate of Parkinson's disease. Numerous studies have shown that those who drink several cups of coffee a day have a lesser chance of developing Parkinson's disease than those who don't drink coffee. In addition, although cigarette smoking is very definitely harmful to health, ironically, people who smoke seem to have lower rates of Parkinson's disease than those who smoke. For reasons that are not clearly understood, nicotine appears to protect the dopamine producing cells in the brain.

This doesn't mean that you should take up smoking, far from it. Like a lot of studies, although the link between smoking and not developing Parkinson's was tenuously established, the fact is that smoking is a killer generally. So, if you don't smoke, don't start.

Diet and nutrition

The exact relationship between diet and nutrition remains, like the other relationships, vague and controversial. Nothing that a person can eat, or not eat, has been definitely linked to

Parkinson's. However, some researchers have shown that diet may help to prevent some cases of the disease. We will be discussing diet later on in the book, but briefly diets rich in antioxidants-such as vitamin C, Vitamin E and Beta-carotene-may help to reduce the levels of free radicals in the body, reducing the risk of developing Parkinson's disease.

Age related factors

In some individuals, the normal age-related wearing away of dopamine producing cells, plus the fact that we are living longer, accelerates the onset of Parkinson's disease. The older you get, whether male or female, the greater the chances of developing Parkinson's disease. The incidence of Parkinson's disease in the under 50's is less than 10 per 100,000 per year compared to more than 200 per 100,000 for those over 80.

In this chapter we have outlined the underlying causes of Parkinson's and also the potential contributory factors. As can be seen, there are a number of factors, however, research hasn't been conclusive and is still carrying on. Age and environmental influences seem to play a major role.

In chapter two we will be looking at the diagnosis of Parkinson's disease and the importance of symptoms in recognising Parkinson's.

****

Chapter 2

The Diagnosis of Parkinson's Disease

As my own experience reflects, the diagnosis of Parkinson's disease has to be carried out very carefully and with certainty, as the consequences of a wrong diagnosis can be very stressful and traumatic for the person involved. In my case, once people, including in the first instance, my doctor, had convinced me that I had Parkinson's disease, I began to prepare myself for a life spent coping with the condition. It is therefore best not to listen to people around you, as everyone seems to be an amateur doctor, but make sure that you have specialist advice.

The main characteristics of Parkinson's disease

Although there are numerous symptoms of Parkinson's disease the main characteristics of include slowness, general stiffness and an ongoing tremor.

Tremor

Tremor, which is the most common symptom associated with Parkinson's disease, is another term for shaking or trembling of the body. There are several types of tremor:

- Rest tremor, which occurs when the limb, usually wrist, fingers or arm, is relaxed and not in use. It ceases when the limb is in use.

- Postural tremor, which occurs when an arm or leg is held out against gravity, such as when holding a newspaper or book.
- Action tremor, as the name suggest this occurs when the limb is in use, such as when preparing food or eating.
- Pill rolling tremor, which occurs when rolling the thumb against the index finger.

Rigidity

Rigidity is a tightening or stiffening of the muscles. There are two basic types of rigidity, lead –pipe rigidity (the body wont move and is stiff, like a lead-pipe) and cogwheel rigidity (the body moves in a jerky motion, similar to the cogs in a wheel). In both types of rigidity the body does not move smoothly and there can also be pain.

The incidence of rigidity and overall stiffness will vary with individuals. Typically, rigidity occurs more on one side that the other and involves arms, legs, neck and back.

Bradykinesia

Bradykinesia is a general term referring to slowness of movement or speech. The term akinesia refers to absence of movement, which can also be a sign of Parkinson's disease. In most cases, akinesia shows up as an arm that does not swing when you walk or similar inability to move voluntarily.

Most people with Parkinson's disease experience some kind of bradykinesia, which can be experienced in a number of ways- from freeze attacks to difficulty dressing and walking to difficulty swallowing. These symptoms will come and go but when they are active the person may feel weakness.

Balance

Another very common symptom of Parkinson's disease is postural instability or problems with balance. Whilst this is not considered to be one of the major symptoms, many people with Parkinson's do have problems with their balance.

There are a number of other symptoms associated with Parkinson's such as light-headedness or fainting, problems with vision, problems with walking, weight loss, sleep problems and urinary problems. This list isn't exhaustive but your doctor, when assessing you for Parkinson's, or initially assessing your condition to determine whether or not it is Parkinson's will take them all into account.

The process of elimination

There is no specific diagnostic procedure or laboratory test to establish the diagnosis of Parkinson's disease. Therefore, a diagnosis is based on patterns. As the disease develops gradually, it is hard to be sure of a diagnosis until enough symptoms are present. Diagnosis is especially difficult in older people, because aging can cause some of the same problems as Parkinson's disease, such as loss of balance, slow movements, muscle stiffness and stooped posture.

Although there are no specific tests for Parkinson's disease, certain types of scans can provide evidence to support clinical diagnosis by measuring the ability of the brain to produce dopamine. These scans use processes called Positron Emission Tomography (PET) or Single Photon Emission Tomography (SPECT). These scans, however, are not used as a standard diagnostic test for Parkinson's disease.

In my own case, I underwent a deep brain scan, which was an unpleasant experience, and it was this scan which provided conclusive evidence that my condition wasn't Parkinson's.

Carrying out the diagnosis

Given the difficult task of initially detecting Parkinson's disease, doctors usually have to carry out detective work, which is, essentially, a three-step process.

1. Assessing the symptoms

To diagnose Parkinson's disease, a doctor-preferably a neurologist or specialist-must carry out a review of the patients detailed medical history and perform a complete physical examination. The doctor will consider all the Parkinson's symptoms. In many cases, doctors will not consider Parkinson's as a possibility if there is not a tremor. However, as one in three people do not have tremors this is not really a very good starting point.

2. Consider all the possible diagnosis

After a detailed study of your symptoms, your doctor will need to look at the possibility of other diseases aside from Parkinson's. In the early stages, it can be very difficult to distinguish. Is arthritis present? Do you have a benign tremor? What exactly is happening? To make this determination, doctors should consider the fact that you may have another condition with symptoms similar to Parkinson's. There are a number of other possibilities:

Aging-this is the most obvious one. People tend to slow down as they get older. They walk more deliberately and experience problems with balance and also develop tremors, similar to Parkinson's.

Arthritis-this is another condition which has similarities to Parkinson's. Arthritis involves bone and joint pain, causing inflammation and loss of coordination. However, the symptoms of arthritis differ from Parkinson's in several ways:

- Arthritis is much easier to confirm with blood tests and x-rays.
- Arthritis causes joint pain and not muscle pain, as with Parkinson's
- Parkinson's symptoms don't respond to medication given for arthritis
- Arthritis doesn't cause tremors with muscle tone remaining normal.

Depression-depression can cause slow movement, stooped posture, weight loss and other common symptoms of Parkinson's. In addition, depression coexists alongside Parkinson's, making diagnosis more difficult. We will be discussing depression a little later in the book.

Essential tremor-many people, including medical people, confuse essential tremor with Parkinson tremor. Essential tremor is far more common than Parkinson's disease. People with essential tremor do not exhibit any other symptoms of

Parkinson's disease, such as rigidity or problems with balance. Essential tremor is usually an action tremor that occurs on both sides, left and right while Parkinson's tremor usually appears at rest and only on one side.

Stroke-in some cases people with Parkinson's disease are diagnosed as having suffered a stroke because they present symptoms on one side of the body (this is most common when the person does not experience a tremor). In strokes, symptoms appear very quickly, whereas with Parkinson's they are gradual. The brain scans of people with Parkinson's are normal whereas scans of people with Parkinson's show evidence straight away.

If, after exhaustive tests, Parkinson's is diagnosed, then a course of medication is prescribed to begin to try to establish a balance and rectify the perceived problems. Even at this stage, there is still a lot of uncertainty as Parkinson's disease is notoriously difficult to diagnose. It is only through time, and the onset of the condition, and trials with medication that the condition can be stabilized.

The next chapter deals with medication and the importance of getting the right medication, and also your role in identifying symptoms which in turn helps the doctor develop a successful program for you. Again, this chapter is not exhaustive as only a specialist can arrive at a correct dosage of the appropriate medication.

****

Chapter 3

Medication and Parkinson's

Having been through the initial, often traumatic, stages of the initial diagnosis, it is very necessary for you to build up a detailed knowledge of the type of medication that you will have to take for Parkinson's disease and also the side effects of that medication plus the effects of mixing medication.

In the first instance, if a doctor thinks that Parkinson's disease may be present, then, typically, a trial dose of dopamine-stimulating medication is administered. If, after this initial medication the patients condition improves then he or she is considered to have Parkinson's. If the patient does not improve then the doctor must consider another diagnosis.

Medications

Drugs that are currently in use to treat Parkinson's disease make movement easier and can prolong functions for many years. Overall, medications in use aim to replace, or to mimic, the missing chemical dopamine in the brain. The pharmacological treatment of Parkinson's is quite complex. While, overall, there are a large number of drugs that can be effective, their effectiveness will vary with the patient, the progression of the disease and the length of time that the medication has been used. Related side effects can preclude the use of certain medications, or require the introduction of a new drug to counteract them. Currently, there are five classes of drugs used to treat Parkinson's disease.

Drugs that replace dopamine

One particular drug that helps to replace dopamine is Levodopa (L-dopa) and is the single most effective treatment for the symptoms of Parkinson's disease. L-dopa is a derivative of dopamine, and is converted into dopamine by the brain. Doctors may choose to commence it when symptoms begin, or when they become serious enough to interfere with work or daily living.

L-dopa therapy usually remains effective for five years or longer. Following this, many patients develop motor fluctuations, including what is known as peak-dose dyskinesias (abnormal movements such as tics, twisting or restlessness) rapid loss of response after dosing and unpredictable drug response. Higher doses are usually tried, but may lead to an increase in dyskinesias. In addition, side effects of L-dopa may be nausea and vomiting, plus low blood pressure which can cause dizziness. These effects usually lessen after several weeks of therapy.

Enzyme inhibitors

Dopamine is broken down by several enzyme systems in the brain and elsewhere in the body and blocking these enzymes is a key strategy to prolonging the effect of a dose of dopamine. The two most commonly prescribed forms of L-dopa contain a drug to limit the amino acid and decarboxylase (an ADC inhibitor), one type of enzyme that breaks down dopamine. These combination drugs are Sinemet and Madopar. Controlled release formulations also aid in prolonging the effective interval of an L-dopa dose. The enzyme Moncamine oxidase B (MAO-B) inhibitor selegiline may be given as an add-on therapy for L-Dopa. Research indicates that selegiline may have a neuroprotective effect, sparing nigral cells from damage by free radicals. Because of this, and the fact that it has few side effects, it is also frequently prescribed early on in the disease before L-Dopa is begun.

Dopamine agonists

Dopamine works by stimulating receptors on the surface of corpus striatum cells. Drugs which also stimulate these receptors are called dopamine agonists. Dopamine agonists are used both as adjuncts to levodopa therapy, and also initially in early Parkinson's disease, especially in young adults. The side effects of dopamine agonists are similar to those of levdopa, although they are less likely to cause involuntary movements and more likely to cause hallucinations or sleepiness.

This class of drugs includes the older dopamine agonists bromocripline (Partodel) and pergolide (permax) and the newer drugs pramipexole (Mirapex) and ropinirole (Requip). You should avoid dopamine agonists if you already experience hallucinations or confusion.

Anticholinergic drugs

Anticholinergics help control tremors in the early stages of the disease. Even so, they are only mildly beneficial and sometimes the benefits are offset by side effects such as dry mouth, nausea, urine retention, especially in men with enlarged prostrate-and severe constipation. These drugs can also cause or exacerbate mental problems, including memory loss, confusion and hallucinations.

Amantadine

Amantadine (Symadine, Symmeterel) stimulates the release of dopamine and may be used for patients with early mild symptoms. It has some benefit against muscle rigidity and slowness and may help older patients who are unresponsive to other drugs. It is less powerful than levodopa and may lose its effectiveness after about six months. It may also reduce motor fluctuations brought on by levadopa.

Using medications safely

There are basic guidelines for safe use of medication, listed below.

- Always continue with your course of medication and don't stop taking it unless you have consulted with your doctor. Appendix one shows an example of a medication log which should always be maintained so that you can produce evidence to your doctor if the medication is, in your opinion, not having the desired effect.
- Always begin medication with the lowest possible dose and increase gradually.
- If you experience side effects from Levdopa treatment ask your doctor about lowering the dose of the drug and adding a dopamine agonist.
- When changing a medication allow two to four weeks for your body to adjust before deciding that it is having a beneficial effect. It can take several weeks for your system to adjust to the new medication or dosage.
- Stick to a regular medication schedule, most important as keeping a steady amount of medication in your system will help reduce the likelihood of motor fluctuations.

- Before you take any new medication, ask your doctor to review the existing medications that you are taking and make sure that there are no side effects from mixing drugs.

The approach to treatment, and the administering of medications, differs for younger and older people. As a general rule, people over the age of 70 tend to take levdopa. Older people have trouble tolerating dopamine agonists without suffering side-effects, including confusion and hallucinations.

Younger people often use dopamine agonists to manage their symptoms early in the disease, in part because younger people experience fewer side effects from these drugs than older people. In addition, younger people often have more time ahead of them to manage Parkinson's symptoms, and many of the drugs will eventually lose their effectiveness.

Whatever the combination of medication used, stay in control, make sure that you medicate regularly and always request information about drugs that you are using, particularly combinations of drugs.

In the next chapter, we will look at current surgery for Parkinson's disease and also at the ongoing research.

****

Chapter 4

Surgery for Parkinson's and Ongoing research

Surgery for Parkinson's Disease

Over the years, surgery for Parkinson's has developed and improved, particularly so since the 1980's. While medication remains the first line of treatment, there are surgical options available which should also be considered. Deep Brain Stimulation is the more common form of surgery used on people with Parkinson's along with what is know as 'lesioning'.

Deep Brain Stimulation

In the late 1990's, deep brain stimulation revolutionized the surgical treatment of Parkinson's disease. The surgery involves inserting a thin wire and electrodes into the brain, linking the wire to a remote battery, and stimulating the brain at a high frequency. The electrodes are positioned in the brain; the wires run under the skin along the skull and down the neck, eventually crossing over to a pacemaker battery pack in the chest wall.

Deep Brain Stimulation does not reverse all the symptoms, but tends to improve symptoms to a level where they were several years before. The physical changes associated with DBS are determined by the positioning of the electrodes.

Lesioning-Pallidotomy and Thalamotomy

Lesioning involves using a heat sensitive probe to make a small hole in the brain that will alter motor function and relieve Parkinson's symptoms.

Pallidotomy

Pallidotomy is the most common lesioning surgery for Parkinson's disease and has been available for the last 50 years. This procedure can help relieve tremors, rigidity and bradykinesia (slowness of movement) by 15-20% and dyskinesia (abnormal movements other than tremor) by up to 80%. However, Pallidotomy doesn't help people with walking and balance. Pallidotomy is often recommended for people with Parkinson's symptoms that cannot be controlled with medication, as well as for those with disabling dyskinesia.

Thalamotomy

Thalamotomy can help reduce Parkinson's tremor and essential tremor by as much as 90% but does not significantly reduce rigidity or bradykinesia. For this reason, thalamotomy is typically used only on patients with tremor-predominant PD or severe essential tremor that does not respond to medication.

Cell implants

Research is under way to find a way to restore function to patients with Parkinson's disease by implanting cells into the damaged region of the brain. Cells from a patient's adrenal medulla (which normally produces neurotransmitter substances including dopamine) have been tried but little improvements in symptoms was found.

Mixed results have been obtained with cells taken from the brain of human foetuses. These cells develop into neurons of the type lost from the substantia nigra in Parkinson's disease. This is a very sensitive and intricate procedure and the results have been varied

Work is now taking place to develop human cells that can be grown in a laboratory and will produce dopamine, perhaps by altering the cells DNA. These cells may then be put into a special type of capsule that protects them but allows the dopamine to leave These capsules may be microscopic and suitable for inserting into the same area of the brain as foetal implants.

Stem cells from embryos

A further area of research is the use of stem cells from human embryos. These cells are at an immature, early stage of development and, with the correct genetic signal, can change into any type of cell, including nerve cells. This is what happens normally after fertilisation-the few cells that grow from the fertilised egg go on to develop into all the different types of cell that form a baby. Each cell in your body has the genetic information to become any type of cell, it just depends which genes are active. It is hoped that we can find out how to switch on the genes that convert stem cells into neurons for implantation to improve Parkinson's disease. This particular research is still at the early stage.

Growth factors

Growth factors are molecules that can be obtained from a variety of different cell types in the body. They occur naturally and are designed to encourage the growth and maturation of cells. Growth factors derived from the brain and glial cells (a type of cell in the brain) have both been used with success sin animals and some Parkinson's disease patients. This research is still in the early stages but may become a useful treatment in the future.

Surgery is one option for people with Parkinson's disease. However, most people try to stabilise the condition with medication. This involves a relationship between you and your doctor. Establishing a strong relationship is of the utmost importance. This relationship must be characterized by trust and openness and also the sharing of information.

In appendix one I have inserted a medication log, which is the main way of compiling ongoing evidence which will inform the doctor and enable him or her to provide the best course of medication. The next chapter deals with your relationship with your doctor and also any specialists that you may see.

Chapter 5

Finding the Right GP/Consultant

It is a fact that many of us will place ourselves in the hands of our doctor's, or consultants, and implicitly trust them to look after us and give us the best advice possible. I am afraid that this is not always borne out by experience. The type of care and advice that you might receive very much depends on the attitudes of individual doctors, some of whom are better than others.

Whether you are in the process of confirming a diagnosis of Parkinson's or need to work with your doctor to manage your ongoing condition, it is absolutely essential that you choose a doctor that you feel comfortable with and that you trust. Normally, within a family doctor practice there are different doctors who tend to specialise. You must ensure that you find the doctor best suited to you. If you have any questions about your diagnosis be sure to seek a second opinion-don't just rely on the diagnosis and 'grin and bear' it. Don't feel afraid to change your doctor if you need to, it is your life and your well-being.

Right at the outset, you will want to identify a group of people who will support you through your condition. These will include:

- A general practitioner, i.e. your doctor, who will address your overall health care and needs and also provide referrals.

- From your doctor's recommendation, a neurologist, who will manage your Parkinson's disease
- A movement-disorders specialist if your neurologist doesn't have experience in this field. The neurologist will usually recommend such a person
- A physical therapist who will help you to develop an exercise regime suited to you
- A dietitian who will assist you with your diet.

It will be up to you to be proactive when establishing this group-you should take the initiative don't leave this to the professionals. My own experience has been that unless you ask you won't always get!

Of most importance, you will want people who have the most experience in treating people with Parkinson's disorders. This is essential. Never be afraid to ask questions about your condition, don't get sidetracked and make sure that you get the right answers. This is particularly the case with medication as, in the first throes of Parkinson's, medication can take some getting used to, with all sorts of side effects. It is this area that you will need to ensure that you get right.

These are a few questions that you might want to ask a doctor:

- Do you have experience of working with Parkinson's patients?
- How many patients do you see on a regular basis?
- What is your personal opinion about surgery for Parkinson's?

- What is the success rate using surgery?
- What is your opinion about alternative therapies?
- Who will cover for you if you are away and I have problems?

One final tip is to always, if possible, try to maintain a record of your symptoms. See the appendix for a sample log. This will ensure that you can demonstrate clearly to the doctor what exactly the problems are.

Always keep a record of the medications that you are using and bring this to the doctors with you. Whilst it is true that the doctor will also have records it is important that you are in control as well as the doctor.

If you feel that it is necessary you should also bring a friend or carer to the doctors appointment with you as they can provide clarification and support. When you are with the doctor, you should not wait for the doctor to ask you about your most pressing concerns but you should outline these concerns right at the outset. Although doctor's are qualified they don't know everything and the dialogue between you and your doctor is a two way process. Tell the doctor everything, even the most embarrassing symptoms that you would rather keep to yourself. It is very important to ensure that he or she has a clear picture of what is happening.

In the next chapter, we will look at the onset of depression and how it affects people with Parkinson's and how to combat it. I have also outlined a number of groups which play an important role in supporting people with Parkinson's.

Chapter 6

Combating Depression

Parkinson's and depression

When a person is diagnosed with Parkinson's, the trauma of that diagnosis can easily lead to depression. It is also common for depression to stay with a person, on and off, for many years. As depression can be debilitating it is very important that you learn to recognise it and handle it to minimise the impact.

Factors contributing to depression

Living with Parkinson's means living with a situation where you are no longer functioning as you were. It is difficult to do the things that you once did and the knowledge that the condition is degenerative also has a negative impact. In addition, your brain chemistry has altered causing biochemical depression.

There are certain warning signs indicating clinical depression, as distinct to the common form of sadness felt by many Parkinson's sufferers.

- Changes in sleep patterns can be an early warning sign
- Changes in weight or eating habits
- Chronic fatigue or ongoing tiredness
- Apathy-although this is often a by product of Parkinson's and can be distinct from depression
- Inability to concentrate or think clearly

- Withdrawal or isolation
- Anger and irritability
- Frequent crying
- Thoughts of suicide
- Apprehension about the future.

For most people with Parkinson's, depression is an organic illness involving both physical and biochemical changes in the body. It is very important to get the right medication at the early stages to minimise these changes. It is also crucial to ensure that you have access to counselling and professional care.

When it comes to treating depression, most mental health professionals rely on three specific forms of treatment, counselling or talking cures, medication (drug therapy) and, in the most extreme cases, ECT or Electro-Convulsive therapy. Usually, a combination of counselling and medication is used in the first instance and has the greatest success rate.

In most cases, depression usually responds relatively quickly to medication, such as drugs that inhibit the reuptake of seretonin (SSRI's) allowing the seretonin in the body to work longer. If you are in medication for depression you need to allow time for the drugs to work. Anti-depressants often take several weeks to lift the symptoms of depression. Medication should be used for several months during an initial period. You should work with your doctor to explore a range of treatments, until you find one suitable for you.

The importance of acceptance of Parkinson's
When people are first diagnosed with Parkinson's, they almost always go through a process of grieving. It is essential that, during

this period, you allow yourself to ride the emotional roller coaster associated with grieving. The five stages of grieving that have been identified are:

- Denial and isolation
- Anger
- Bargaining
- Depression
- Acceptance

Acceptance is the stage that you want to arrive at but you won't get there unless you have travelled through the other stages. The ongoing challenge with Parkinson's disease is that, once you have reached the stage of acceptance, you experience another setback or new symptoms that may require you to start the process over again. However, once you have reached the stage of acceptance then you will almost certainly be resilient enough to carry on.

It is very difficult indeed, in practice, to remain stoic when you are experiencing the ongoing conditions associated with Parkinson's. It is also very difficult for partners or those around you. The most important element here is having a knowledge of the condition and a future, forward looking philosophy that will take you through the dark times and allow you to focus on the future.

The importance of support groups

In the light of what we have just discussed, and the fact that most peoples personal circumstances differ, some have family, children and grandchildren, parents and so on, some people have no one, it is very important that people with Parkinson's have access to support groups. Within support groups you can share experiences and begin to understand that you are not alone with the condition. You can form new friendships and also gain invaluable advice about day-to-day living.

You will find many useful addresses at the rear of the book which can point you in the right direction, particularly in your own area. One of the first ports of call is Parkinson's UK, formerly the Parkinson's Disease Society, address and website below and at the back of the book. This organisation provides a wealth of information and advice and guidance about Parkinson's disease. Below are some of the groups in alphabetical order and which are repeated in the back of the book.

European Parkinson's Disease Association
(EPDA)
4 Golding Road
Sevenoaks
Kent
TN13 3NJ
Tel: 01732 457683
www.epda.eu.com

Umbrella body for network of international
Parkinson's disease groups, campaigning on behalf
Of all suffers. Information leaflets on request.
An S.A.E. requested.

Leonard Cheshire
66 South Lambeth Road
London
SW8 1RL

Tel: 020 3242 0200
www.lcdisability.org
Email: info@lcdisability.org
Offers care, support and a wide range of
Information for disabled people aged between
18 and 65 years in the UK and worldwide to
encourage independent living. Has respite
and residential homes; offers holidays
and rehabilitation.

Parkinson's UK
National Office
215 Vauxhall Bridge Road
London
Hepline: 0808 800 0303
Tel: 020 7931 8080
Fax: 020 7233 9908
www.parkinsons.org.uk
Offers information and support via its local groups
Has nurse specialists and welfare department,
And funds research into Parkinson's disease.

Patients' Association
PO Box 935
Harrow
Middlesex
HA1 3YJ
Helpline: 0845 608 4455
Tel: 020 8423 9111
www.patients-association.com
Email: helpline@patients-association.com

Provides advice on patients' rights, leaflets and also a directory of
self-help groups.

RADAR: The Disability Network
12 City Forum
250 City Road
London
EC1V 8AF
Tel: 020 7250 3222
Minicom: 020 7250 4119
www.radar.org.uk
Email: radar@radar.org.uk
Campaigns to improve the rights and care of
Disabled people. Sells special key to access locked disabled toilets.

Vitalise (previously Winged Fellowship Trust)
12 City Forum
250 City Road
London
EC1V 8AF
Tel: 0845 345 1972
Fax: 0845 345 1978
www.vitalise.org.uk
Offers holidays at their own centres and overseas
And respite care for people with severe disabilities by
Prviding voluntary carers. Also arrages holidays for
People with Alzheimer's disease/dementia and
Their carers.

YPN (Younger Parkinson's Network)
National helpline : 0808 800 0303
www.http://yap-web.net

The young-onset self-help group of the Parkinson's
Disase Society and is designed really for those of
Working age. There are around 1,300 members
Of YPN , many of them in their early 20s and 30s.
Has a magazine, local meetings and conference every
2 years.

David Rayner Centre
120 Cambridge Road
Great Shelford
Cambridege
CB22 5JT
Helpline: 080 8800 0303
www.parkinsons.org.uk

Network of local groups bringing people
With Parkinson's and their families
Together for support and help.

Parkinson's Home Care
Helping Hand Homecare
Arrow House
8-9 Church Street
Alcester
Warwickshire
B49 5AJ
Free phone: 0808 180 9455
www.helpinghandscare.co.uk

Support Group for Asian People
Valley Gardens
West Bridgford

Nottingham
NG2 6HG
Email: mkraca@kaura.me-uk

Although specific to Nottingham this group can offer general advice to Asian people.

One of the most invaluable resources available to you is the internet. You can locate support groups local to you by surfing the web. In addition, Libraries are invaluable sources of information.

In the next chapter, we will move on to discussing the importance of diet and nutrition for those with Parkinson's. Many of the tips are universal and are common sense to all people. However, they are particularly important for those with Parkinson's.

Chapter 7

Diet and Parkinson's Disease

Whilst there is no special diet in use for people with Parkinson's disease, as with all people a well-balanced nutritious diet is an absolute must and will, in the long term, prove beneficial. It is a well-known fact that with a proper diet, our bodies work more efficiently and we feel a lot more healthy. The upshot of this is that Parkinson's disease medications will work properly and more effectively with a well-balanced diet.

We (the authors) are not specialist dietitians and make no recommendations based on any specialism. The information contained below is based on good common sense and information gleaned from specialist publications.

Eating well with Parkinson's

Generally, Parkinson's patients should eat a well balanced diet, high in fruits and vegetables and relatively low in protein. The following represents sound guidelines for people with PD.

It is generally accepted that people with Parkinson's should eat more fibre. This helps to prevent constipation and helps to speed food through the digestive tract, minimising the amount of time that food remains in the intestines. Most people eat about 15 grams of fibre daily. Those with Parkinson's should strive to eat about double that amount. A useful source of fibre is dried fruit. You should also switch from refined to whole grains. You may also want to consider fibre supplements. Add these supplements to your diet slowly to avoid side effects which can include gas or diarrhoea.

In addition, it helps if Parkinson's sufferers drink lots of water. This helps with constipation and also helps with the respiratory system, acts as a lubricant and flushes waste through the bloodstream. It is a fact that some Parkinson's medication can contribute to dehydration. A good daily intake of water is around eight 8-ounce glasses per day. This should, ideally, be filtered or bottled water.

It is also well worth considering probiotics, or yoghurt. The 'good' bacteria found in yoghurt with live cultures and supplements help complete the digestive process, reduce inflammation and balance the endocrine system. You can obtain such foods from good health food stores and also pharmacies.

Like a lot of people with any sort of condition, it is best to avoid spicy foods. Some people with Parkinson's find that they experience violent dyskinesia after they eat spicy foods. It is best to give such foods a miss.

It is a fact that people with Parkinson's can be susceptible to thinning bones caused by osteoporosis. Foods high in calcium, magnesium and vitamin D should be consumed, timed to complement your medication.

The maintenance of a healthy weight is very important and you will need to watch your calorie intake so that you can maintain your ideal weight. Some people with Parkinson's will lose weight (tremors and dyskinesia can burn an excessive amount of calories) others will gain weight as a result of the side effects of some medications).

Underweight

You may find that you are underweight and have difficulty putting weight on. Sometimes, weight loss can be due to practical problems to do with food preparation and keeping your food hot while you are eating.

The way you buy, store, prepare and cook food may need a little rethinking. It is recommended that you seek advice from an occupational therapist who can advise you on all aspects of food shopping and preparation, including kitchen and shopping aids. Here are a few tips:

- You should always try to plan your meals in advance, making a shopping list of all the necessary ingredients.
- When you are planning meals, you should decide how long you should stand at a cooker before you get tired.
- You should consider buying foods that are already prepared, such as frozen foods like vegetables and tinned fish, meat or beans. Ready meals will save time on all fronts.
- Keep well stocked with a wide supply of food.
- If you can, purchase a microwave, as they will save a lot of time.

- If you like a nap in the afternoon, keep hot water in a flask on a tray with a tea bag, milk, sugar etc. Drinking regularly helps you to keep warm
- You may be entitled to meals on wheels or home delivery of frozen meals. You should contact the home care organiser of your local social services department.

Dishes and cutlery

There are a variety of adapted utensils for eating and drinking which may be worth buying. However, it is strongly recommended that you seek the advice of an occupational therapist before buying expensive specialised equipment.

Specialised cutlery is available in various shapes and sizes and you should use large mugs for drinks, but only half full. Two-handled cups can improve grip and reduce the chance of spillage. Special 'tumble-not' mugs are available with wide, non-slip bases and tall necks.

A 'stay-warm' plate might be useful if it takes you a long time to eat, or you could have smaller, more frequent meals. A damp cloth placed under a plate will stop it from slipping, or special mats can be used. High lipped plates are available that prevent spillage and make it easier to draw food onto the fork or spoon. Similarly, plate guards can be bought that clip onto your usual plates. Equipment is also available to help with opening jars and bottles. Information on all of the above specialist equipment can be obtained from Parkinson's UK.

Advice on eating and swallowing food

As important as diet, and the preparation of food, is how you eat. The following tips might be helpful:

- Take your time when you eat. Eat in a comfortable, quiet setting. However, if you feel that you are taking too long and your food is getting cold, consider eating smaller more frequent meals, or food that is easier to eat.
- Try eating in the recommended eating position. This is sitting upright in a chair with both feet on the floor and the arm that you are not using resting on the table.
- Try planning your meals for when your medication is working. You should avoid eating large meals when you are off your medication.
- Some people feel their throats tense up while eating and food sticks in their throat. You should try yawning before a meal to relax your throat.

Some people find certain foods more difficult to chew or swallow than others. If this is the case then you may want to consider a semi-solid diet. However, before you do so, you should speak to a registered dietitian or your GP who can advise you. This is because not all swallowing problems are to do with Parkinson's and it is necessary to confirm the cause of the problem before changing diet. You can also be advised on the best consistency and texture of food/liquid for you.

Semi-solid foods are generally easier to swallow than foods with mixed textures or very hard or dry foods.

Tips on easier swallowing:

- Try slightly thicker creamy soups rather than watery ones, or those with 'bits' in.
- Meat that is tough or chewy can be difficult. Try moistening this with either gravy or some kind of sauce, or try fish, which is usually softer.
- Try mashed potato, pasta or noodles as a change from bread.
- Try wholemeal instead of white bread as white bread can get stuck in the mouth.
- Try soft, moist biscuits, such as sponge fingers rather than drier crackers or toast.
- Having a drink with your meal makes chewing softer. Iced water in particular may help the 'strength' of your swallow.
- Good posture and a comfortable position when eating will also aid swallowing.
- Try taking smaller mouthfuls.
- If you wear dentures make sure that they fit properly.

Puree diets

If you find swallowing very difficult, you should again seek advice from suitably qualified people, such as a GP, dietitian or therapist. They might suggest that you try a puree diet. Below are some tips on a puree diet.

- If foods are being liquidised or pureed, always use a milk based sauce or gravy, rather than water. This will increase the nutrients and energy of the meal.

- Do not use baby foods; although they may be the right texture, they are not nutritionally adequate for adults.
- Thickening agents can be added to liquidised or pureed foods to add back some of the texture. Suitable thickeners include milk powder, instant potato powder, custard powder or plain yoghurt.

Speech and language therapists, occupational therapists and registered dietitians can also advise further on diet, utensils and eating techniques. Again, there is plenty of information on the web site of Parkinson's UK related to diet.

A sample eating plan

As has been outlined above, and is also common sense, good nutrition in Parkinson's involves eating regularly, and also eating a wide range of different foods. Below is a sample eating plan with a variety of foods from which you can choose. Please bear in mind that this is only a sample and that you should pick and choose from what has been outlined.

Breakfast	Fruit or fruit juice; cereal and milk; bread toast and butter (or margarine, soya spread etc) eggs, bacon, sausage etc; tea, coffee or milk.
Midday meal:	Meat, fish, eggs or cheese or alternative(consider cholesterol) Potato, rice, pasta or bread/toast;vegetables, yoghurt, custard or fruit drink.
Evening meal	Soup of fruit juice; meat, fish,

	eggs, beans or lentils, potato, rice, pasta, bread: salad or vegetables, yoghurt, ice cream and jelly
Between meals	Have a drink between meals, as well as with them, for example tea, coffee, soup, fruit juice, water etc. You can also smack lightly.
The main meals, midday and evening are interchangeable.	

Parkinson's medication and the interaction with food

Each of the medications in use with Parkinson's disease has a particular interaction with food. For example, levdopa generally works better when taken on an empty stomach. Therefore your doctor may possibly prescribe a combination of levdopa and carbidopa (known as sinemet) or carbidopa by itself (called Lodosyn). If nausea is a continual problem, then another drug may be prescribed to relieve these symptoms.

Controlling nausea

Given that nausea can be a problem with Parkinson's patients, it is useful to understand the best ways to control nausea. The following are useful tips:

- Drink clear or ice cold drinks. Drinks containing a small amount of sugars may calm the stomach better than other liquids.

- Avoid acidic drinks such as orange or grapefruit juices as they may worsen nausea.

- Drink liquids in between meals instead of during them.

- Avoid fried, greasy foods (always best avoided in all circumstances).

- Eat slowly, don't bolt food and eat smaller more frequent portions instead of large meals.

- Don't mix hot and cold foods. Eat foods that are cold at room temperature.

- Rest after you eat, don't rush around as this will bring on nausea.

Vitamins and minerals

Eating a well-balanced diet will provide adequate levels of vitamins and minerals for most people. Food contains fibre and other valuable nutrients, as well as vitamins and minerals. Essentially, if you feel that you are in need of more of a particular vitamin or mineral, it is usually advised that you eat more of the particular food containing them rather than buying expensive supplements.

In the next chapter, we will look at the benefits of exercise and Parkinson's disease. Exercise compliments diet and the two can combine to make you a healthy and able to cope better with life and your condition.

Chapter 8

The Benefits of Exercise and Parkinson's

Most people with Parkinson's understand the importance of exercise in the control and improvement of the disease.

Research has shown that there are several types of muscle weakness involved with Parkinson's, including weakening of the pulmonary muscles. Although those with Parkinson's will find it difficult at times to carry out exercises, it is important that a regular regime is adhered to.

The benefits of exercise

Exercise offers significant health benefits for everyone, whether or not they have Parkinson's disease. Exercise improves emotional and physical health, reduces risk of serious illness and increases overall energy levels. For those with Parkinson's regular exercise can help improve flexibility, reduce muscle stiffness and slow the advancement of Parkinson's symptoms.

Putting together an exercise plan

A well-rounded exercise plan includes three main components: aerobic fitness, muscle strength and flexibility.

Aerobic fitness

The word *Aerobic'* means 'using oxygen'. During aerobic exercise, your heart and lungs work harder than normal to provide muscles with the oxygen they demand, and you breath heavily and steadily to meet your body's increased need for oxygen. During an aerobic exercise, your heart and lungs cannot meet your body's increased need for oxygen for longer than a minute or two, and you are left gasping for breath, even if you are in fairly good condition. Simple aerobic exercises include jogging and running short distances.

Jogging and running may not be everyone's idea of fun and there are alternatives to this. Swimming is a very good exercise as are other forms of gym exercise. The important thing is to find an exercise that is suitable for your condition and temperament.

Numerous studies have found that aerobic exercise not only helps people with Parkinson's disease improve their aerobic capacity, but it also helps with movement problems, such as freezing.

When choosing an aerobic activity, you need to find an exercise that involves the rhythmic, repeated use of the major muscle groups, such as walking, yoga, or tai chi. When done regularly-for example three times a week for at least 20-30 minutes at a time-aerobic exercises improve the efficiency of the heart, lungs and muscles.

To derive the maximum benefit from these exercises, you need to work hard enough, but not too hard, particularly in the beginning and also if you need to lose some weight. You need to ease in slowly but surely. Your pulse rate (heart beats per minute) is your body's speedometer. It tells you how fast your heart is going and if you need to speed up or slow things down. Cardiovascular conditioning takes place when your heart beats at 70-85 per cent of its maximum safe rate. Your maximum heart rate is approximately 220 minus your age.

Dancing or exercising to music is seen as beneficial. Studies have found that people with Parkinson's disease who participated in music therapy-including rhythmic and free body movement-experienced significant reduction in bradykinesia (slowness of movement and rigidity).

In addition to regular workouts, it is important that Parkinson's sufferers remain as active as possible at all times. This can involve any type of activity, such as shopping, walking around the garden or playing with children or grandchildren.

Improving muscle strength

Whilst Parkinson's sufferers are prone to muscle weakness and atrophy, they are not particularly side effects of Parkinson's or inevitable effects of aging. However, they do happen and there is only one way to combat this and that is through exercise. You can keep muscles strong and supple by performing strength-building exercises, such as weightlifting and isometric exercises.

Strength training also helps stabilize the joints and reduce risks of falling and injury. It has been proven that strength training also helps people with Parkinson's disease improve their walking velocity and stride length. Since most people with Parkinson's disease have some trouble with walking or gait at some time, it is clear that some type of strength training should be some part of your exercise programme.

Without strength training, you will lose muscle mass and strength. The average person will lose 10-20 percent of muscle strength between the ages of 20 to 50, and then another 25 to 30% between 50 to 70. However, this can be held at bay, or slowed, by strength training.

Flexibility

Flexibility is the opposite of rigidity, which is one of the defining characteristics of Parkinson's disease. Flexibility involves maintaining the range of motion in your joints, which can allow you to perform your everyday activities without discomfort. Maintaining flexibility makes you less prone to muscle strains and sprains, and helps you support your joints.

Stretching is the key to preserving your flexibility. Begin with 10-minute stretching sessions in the morning and evening and work your way towards 20-minute sessions twice a day. You should move and stretch your entire body-neck, shoulders, waist, fingers, wrists, elbows, arms, toes, ankles, legs and hips-through their full range of motion in every direction. You should gently stretch and hold, then repeat two or three times. Only stretch to levels that you are comfortable with, don't overstretch as this can make things worse.

Stretch your facial muscles by opening your jaw, raise eyebrows, smile make facial expressions. Try to massage your face gently to reach the tiny muscles in your face. You need to talk to your GP or a therapist about a full list of stretching exercises, as you should for all other exercises.

Starting your exercises

For some people, it might be better to get a partner to help them begin exercising. This can be for the pleasure of exercising with someone else and also for practical reasons, such as someone to help you with balance and to assist you if you fall over. A very good option is to join a local group at a community centre or clinic. This might motivate you to maintain continuity. You can also share experiences.

Never do more than you can manage and never do any exercise that causes pain. You don't want to pull muscles or irritate joints.

Organisations such as Parkinson's UK can give guidance on various forms of exercise and offer recommended programmes of exercise.

The next chapter deals with the range of welfare benefits available for people with Parkinson's (although many are also relevant to everyone). For many, as the condition progresses, benefits and general support will play a vital role in their lives.

Chapter 9

Welfare Benefits and Employment

This chapter, which may seem laborious, contains essential information about the types of benefits available to Parkinson's sufferers and their carers. Whilst in the first instance, benefits may not be of great importance to a person with early stage Parkinson's, as time goes on they will grow in importance so it is beneficial to have a fairly detailed knowledge of what is on offer.

The below lists all the main benefits on offer.

Whilst this chapter may seem exhaustive it is necessary to cover all benefits in detail. We will start with disability benefits as these are likely to play an important role in life as time goes on.

Disability Living Allowance

If you are under the age of 65 and need help looking after yourself or find it difficult to get around then you will probably be entitled to Disability Living Allowance. The allowance has two parts, the care component and the mobility component (the government is currently looking at the provision of these and a wider range of benefits but the information below is correct at the time of going to print).

The care component

This will be applicable to you if you need help looking after yourself or if you need someone around to make sure that you are safe. This component has three rates and the rate depends on the amount of care or supervision that you need.

Care Component	Weekly Rates
Highest rate	£73.60 (2011-12)
Middle rate	£49.30
Lowest rate	£19.55

The mobility component

This is paid to people who have problems walking outside their homes. It has two rates and this depends on how severe your condition is.

Mobility Component	Weekly rate
Higher rate	£51.40 (2011-2012)
Lower rate	£19.55

Disability Living Allowance is paid direct to the person needing the care or supervision and not the carer. You don't necessarily need someone looking after you to receive the payment and it is entirely up to you how you use it. This benefit is not means tested and isn't affected by income or savings or National Insurance contributions.

Claiming the allowance

You can claim DLA if you have needed help for three months or longer. You must also be likely to need help for at least six months after your claim. If you want to go ahead and make a claim or want to know more about it you can phone the Benefit Enquiry Line on 0800 882 200 and they will send you one. You can also obtain one online from www.direct.gov/disability-dla

Attendance allowance

If you are over the age of 65 and have an illness or disability, needing help with personal care, or someone to watch over you, then you can claim Attendance Allowance. This again is paid direct to you and you don't need someone looking after you to make a claim.

As with DLA, Attendance Allowance is paid at one of two rates, depending on the help you need, not on the help you actually get. Again, it is not means tested and doesn't depend on National Insurance contributions or any other benefit you might get.

Attendance allowance	Weekly rates
Higher rate	£73.60 (2011-2012)
Lower rate	£49.80

Claiming Attendance Allowance

You will normally only receive Attendance Allowance if you have needed help for six months or longer. To make a claim, you will need to fill in form A1 which you can either request from the Benefits Enquiry Helpline, as above or from the website www.direct.gov.uk/disability-aa

If your condition worsens and you need more care and supervision you can be reassessed and may be entitled to a higher rate of benefit. If you need to be reassessed then you should contact the benefits helpline.

Benefits payable if you cannot work because of illness, disability, age or caring responsibilities

Of the below listed benefits, you can only claim one at any one time. If you qualify for more than one benefit you can claim the one that pays the highest amount.

Statutory Sick pay

Statutory Sick pay is payable to people who are employed but cannot work due to ill health. It is paid by the employer for the first 28 weeks in any one period of sickness. This includes different periods of sickness linked by less than eight weeks. If you have more than one job you may be able to get SSP from each employer.

In order to qualify for SSP you can be employed to work full or part time, have been sick for at least four or more days in a row, including weekends, bank holidays and days that you do not normally work, and must be have been earning an average of at least £102 (Lower Earnings Limit) per week (2011/2012). This is lower than the amount that you would need to earn before you start paying national insurance.

How average earnings are worked out

From April 2011, you must have average earnings of at least £102 a week before National Insurance and tax are deducted. Your average weekly earnings are calculated over the eight weeks before your sickness began. This period may vary slightly depending on whether you are paid weekly, monthly or have other pay patterns. If you have just started your job the calculation may be different. You should contact your employer for more information. Only earnings actually paid in this eight-week period can be used for the average weekly earnings calculation. These earnings must be subject to National Insurance contributions or would be if your earnings were high enough and may include:

- Your normal earnings
- Bonuses
- Holiday pay
- Overtime
- Other statutory payments

Salary sacrifice scheme and SSP

If you have a salary sacrifice arrangement, you average weekly earnings are calculated using the actual earnings (minus the salary sacrifice) paid to you. This could mean that your average weekly earnings may not reach the Lower Earnings Limit for payment of SSP.

Agency workers

If you meet the qualifying conditions for payment, SSP is payable to you. It remains payable while you are working on an assignment or under contract with your agency. Your employer can't end your contract of service to avoid paying you SSP.

This particular benefit is taxable and National Insurance is also deducted. Your employer may pay extra sick pay on top of statutory sick pay. If you are on a low income you may be able to top up your SSP with Income Support or Pension Credit. In order to pay you must inform your employer that you are off sick and also must get a doctor's certificate after seven days sickness.

Statutory sick pay rates

Statutory sick pay 2011-2012	£81.60 per week

Employment and Support Allowance

Employment and Support Allowance (ESA) is a benefit paid if your ability to work is limited by ill health or disability. It is made up of two allowances-Contributory ESA, which has replaced Incapacity Benefit, and Income Related ESA. You may be entitled to either one or both of these allowances.

To get contributory ESA, you will need to have paid enough NI contributions in specified tax years. If you have a limited capability for work and claim ESA before the age of 20 (or 25 if you have been in education or approved training) you do not have to satisfy these contribution conditions. There are no additions for any dependants that you night have.

Income related ESA is a means tested benefit. Your needs are compared with your resources such as income and savings. It can be paid on its own if you are not entitled to contributory ESA and as a top up if you are. Income related ESA can also help towards mortgage costs and certain other housing costs.

To claim ESA call the Jobcentre plus claim line on 0800 055 6688.

An assessment phase of 13 weeks will usually apply to all new ESA claimants, during which time Jobcentre plus will gather information relating to your claim. This involves a Work Capability Assessment, which determines whether you stay on ESA, and what rate it is paid at.

Rates of ESA

Weekly rate during the assessment phase

Single person under 25	Up to £53.45
Single person 25 or over	Up to £67.50

Weekly rate during the main phase

The main phase starts from week 14 of your claim, if the Work Capability Assessment shows that your illness or disability does limit your ability to work.

Type of group	Weekly amount
A single person in the Work Related Activity Group	Up to £94.25
A single person in the Support Group	Up to £99.85

In most cases, you will not get any money for the first three days of your claim. These are called 'waiting days'. Depending on your circumstances, you may be able to get more money if you get income related Employment and Support Allowance. You can only get extra money for your husband, wife or civil partner if you get income related Employment and Support Allowance.

Customers moving onto Employment and Support Allowance from incapacity benefits

If you are moving onto Employment and Support Allowance after the review of your claim to:

- Incapacity benefit
- Income Support paid on the grounds of illness or disability
- Severe Disablement Allowance

you will be told whether you are in the Support Group or Work Related Activity Group.

If the amount of incapacity benefit that you get is more than the amount of Employment and Support Allowance, you will get a top-up payment. The amount of benefit that you get won't rise until the amount of Employment and Support Allowance catches up with the amount of top-up payment.

If the amount of incapacity benefit that you get is lower than the amount of Employment and Support Allowance, you will get more money.

Pension income rules

If you receive contribution-based Employment and Support Allowance and have a gross pension income of more than £85 per week, the amount of benefit payable will be reduced to half the excess. The excess is the difference between £85 and the actual pension income.

If you receive income-related Employment and Support Allowance, any pension income you have will be taken into account, regardless of the amount.

Income tax

Income related Employment and Support Allowance is not taxable.

It is important to note that contribution based Employment and Support Allowance is taxable, so you may have to pay tax. The amount will be dependant on other income you may have and your total income.

The State Pension

Over 96% of single pensioners and 99% of couples receive the basic state pension. Everyone who has paid the appropriate national insurance contributions will be entitled to a state pension. If you are not working you can either receive pension credits, or make voluntary contributions.

The basic state pension is paid at a flat rate, currently for a single person £97.65 per week. For a couple, whether married or not, who have built up their own right to claim the basic pension could receive up to twice this amount £195.30 (2010-11). A married couple can qualify for a higher pension based on the husband's NI contributions. If the wife has reached pension age her part of the pension is paid directly to her. If the wife is below pension age, the whole pension is paid directly to the husband.

Basic state pensions are increased each April in line with price inflation. State pensioners also receive a (£10 Christmas bonus-check current entitlement) and are entitled to winter fuel payments.

At the moment, only married women can claim a pension based on their spouse's NI record. This is set to change and married men who have reached 65 will be able to claim a basic state pension based on their wife's contribution record where the wife reaches state pension age on or after 6th April 2010.

Same sex couples, as a result of the Civil Partnerships Act 2004, have the same rights as heterosexual couples in all aspects of pension provision.

Qualifying for state pension

In order to receive the full basic pension, if you reach state pension age before 6th April 2010 the main rule is that you will have to have paid NI contributions for at least 90% of the tax years in your working life. If you have only paid for a quarter, for example, you may not get basic state pension. 'Working life' is defined as from the age 16 to retirement age, or the last complete tax year before retirement age.

For men and women born after 5th March 1955 the working life is 49 years. For women with a pension age of 60, the working life is 44 years. For NI contributions to count towards a state pension, they must be the right type, as the following table indicates.

NI contributions counting towards a basic state pension.

Type of contribution	Paid by	Details for 2010-11
No Contributions but earnings between LEL and PT	Employees	Earning between 97 and 110 per week
Class 1 full rate on earnings between PT and UAP	Employees	Earnings between 110 and 770. usually paid at 11% but less if contracted out (see further on)
Class 2	Self-employed	Flat rate of 2.40 per week. Those with earnings for the year of less than 5075 can choose to opt out
Class 3	Out of the labour market and not receiving NI credits	Flat rate of 12.05 per week

Key to abbreviations
LEL = Lower earnings limit: PT = Primary Threshold: UAP = Upper Accruals Point: UEL = Upper earnings limit. LEL, PT and UEL usually increase each year UAP is fixed. A rate is due to increase by 1% from 2011-2012 onwards.

National Insurance Contributions that do not count towards the basic state pension.

Type of contribution	Paid By	Details for 2010-11
No Contributions and earnings below the LEL	Employees	Earning less than £97
Class 1, married women's reduced rate	Employees	4.85% of earnings between £110 and £844 per week and 1% above £844 (a)
Class 1, full rate, on earnings above the UAP	Employees	11% of earnings between £770 and £844 per week and 1% on earnings above £844 (a)
No Class 2 contributions	Self-employed	Those with earnings for the year of less than £5,075 who have chosen to opt out
Class 4	Self-employed	8% of earnings for the year between £5,175 and £43,875 and 1% on earnings above £43,875 (a)

Class 1 contributions

Class 1 contributions are paid if earnings are above the primary threshold. The Threshold, set by government annually, is currently £110 per week (tax year 2010/11). If your earnings are above this set limit then you will be paying contributions at class 1 that build up to a state pension.

The level of contribution is set at 11% of earnings above the primary threshold level up to an upper earnings limit which is £844 per week in 2010/11. Contributions are paid at 1% of earnings above the upper earnings limit. If a person earns less than the primary threshold they will not pay NI contributions. The year will still count towards building up a basic state pension provided the earnings are not less than the lower earnings limit. This is £97 at 2010/11.

Class 2 contributions

Self-employed people will build up their NI contributions by paying class 2 contributions. These are paid either by direct debit or by quarterly bill at the rate of £2.40 per week (2010/11).

If profits are below the 'small earnings exception' which is £5075 in 2010/11 then there is a choice of whether or not to pay NI contributions. However, if this option is chosen, then a state pension will not be building up and there could be a loss of other benefits, such as sickness, bereavement and incapacity.

If you are a director of your own company then class 1 contributions will be paid and not class 2.

NI contribution credits

If a person is not working, in some cases they will be credited with NI contributions. This applies in the following circumstances:

- If claiming certain state benefits such as jobseekers allowance, maternity allowance or incapacity benefit
- To men and women under state pension age who have reached 60 but stopped work
- For the years in which a person has had their 16th, 17th or 18th birthday if they were still at school and were born after 5th April 1957.

If a person stays at home in order to look after children or a sick or elderly relative they might qualify for Home Responsibilities Protection. This reduces the number of years of NI contributions that are needed to qualify for a given level of pension. People who are not working and are claiming child benefit will receive Home Responsibilities Protection automatically.

Class 3 contributions

If a person is not paying class 1 or 2 contributions or receiving HRP they can pay class 3 voluntary contributions. These are charged at a flat rate of £12.05 per week (2010/11). They can be paid up to 6 years back to make up any shortfall.

National Insurance Credits

In some situations you may get National Insurance Credits, which plug what would otherwise be gaps in your NI record. You might get credits in the following situations.

- At the start of your working life. For the years in which you had your 16th, 17th and 18th birthdays if you were still at school and were born on or after 6th April 1957. You should get these credits automatically.

- While training. For the years in which you take part in an approved training course if you were born on or after 6th April 1957. Going to university does not count as an approved course. You should normally get these credits automatically.
- When you earn less than the lower earnings limit (£97 per week in 2010-11) and you are claiming working tax credit (or previously Working Families Tax Credit or Disabled person's Tax Credit) you should get these credits automatically.
- While temporarily working abroad if the UK has a reciprocal agreement with the country in which you are working and you are paying contributions there.
- While out of work because of unemployment or illness. If you are claiming job seekers allowance or Employment and Support Allowance, you should get these credits automatically. If you are getting Statutory Sick Pay and the year in which you get it would not otherwise be a qualifying year, you need to claim this credit by writing to the NICO Contributor Group by 31st December following the end of the tax year in which you were on sick leave.
- While you are on maternity (or adoption) leave and receiving Statutory maternity or Adoption Pay and the year in which you get it would not otherwise be a qualifying year. You need to claim this credit by writing to the NICO Contributor Group by 31st December following the end of the tax year in which you were on leave.
- You are a parent of a child under the age of 12 for whom you are getting child benefit. Credits are awarded automatically. You are also eligible if you are a foster

carer, but in that case you will need to claim the carer's credit.

- You are a carer looking after someone with a disability or frail through old age. You get credits automatically if you are claiming Carer's Allowance. Otherwise you will need to make a claim for the Carer's Credit.
- You are on jury service and you earnings are below a certain limit (£97 a week in 2010-11). This applies to the years from 1988-89 onwards. You need to claim this credit by writing to the NICO Contributor Group by 31st December following the end of the tax year in which you were on jury service.
- You are a man under state pension age but older than the state pension age for women. You qualify if you are not paying NI contributions or are already getting credits for some other reason. You do not have to sign on as unemployed and should get these credits automatically.

Women's state pension age is gradually increasing and when it matches the State Pension Age for men from April 2020 onwards, this type of credit will no longer be available.

The State Pension age

Currently, the state pension age is 65 for men. On 6th April 2010, the state pension age for women started to increase gradually from 60-65, to match men's. There will be further increases in the state pension age to 68 for men and women. The increase in the State Pension age is being phased in and your own particular pension age depends on when you were born. The proposed changes affect people born between April 1953 and 5th April 1960. The table below shows the proposed retirement ages.

These changes are not yet law as they need to go to parliament for approval. (For your own retirement age you should go to the Pensions Service Website).

Table 1 indicates proposed pension changes for women.

Table 1.

Date of Birth	Date State pension Age Reached
6th April 1953 to 5th May 1953	6th July 2016
6th May 1953 to 6th June 1953	6th November 2016
6th June 1953 to 5th July 1953	6th March 2017
6th July 1953 to 5th August 1953	6th July 2017
6th August 1953 to 5th September 1953	6th November 2017
6th September 1953 to 5th October 1953	6th March 2018
6th October 1953 to 5th November 1953	6th July 2018
6th November 1953 to 5th December 1953	6th November 2018

Table 2. Indicates proposed changes for men and women

Table 2.

Date of Birth	Date State Pension Age Reached
6th December 1953 to 5th January 1954	6th March 2019
6th January 1954 to 5th February 1954	6th July 2019

6th February 1954 to 5th March 1954	6th November 2019
6th March 1954 to 5th April 1954	6th March 2010
6th April 1954 to 5th April 1960	Your 66th Birthday

State pensions for people over 80

From the age of 80, all pensioners qualify for an extra 25pence per week If a person does not qualify for a basic state pension or is on a low income then they may be entitled to receive what is called ' an over-80's pension' from the age of 80.

For further advice concerning pensions either go to the government website www.thepensionsservice.gov.uk or refer to the list of useful leaflets at the back of this book.

Additional state pension

S2P replaced the State Earnings Related Pension (SERPS) in April 2002. SERPS was, essentially, a state second tier pension and it was compulsory to pay into this in order to supplement the basic state pension. There were drawbacks however, and many people fell through the net so S2P was introduced to allow other groups to contribute. S2P refined SERPS allowing the following to contribute:

- People caring for children under six and entitled to child benefit

- Carers looking after someone who is elderly or disabled, if they are entitled to carers allowance
- Certain people who are unable to work because of illness or disability, if they are entitled to long-term incapacity benefit or severe disablement allowance and they have been in the workforce for at least one-tenth of their working life

Self-employed people are excluded from S2P as are employees earning less than the lower earnings limit. Married women and widows paying class 1 contributions at the reduced rate do not build up additional state pension. S2P is an earnings related scheme. This means that people on high earnings build up more pension than those on lower earnings. However, people earning at least the lower earnings limit (£97) in 2010/11 but less than the low earnings threshold (£110) in 2010/11 are treated as if they have earnings at that level and so build up more pension than they otherwise would.

Contracting out

A person does not build up state additional pension during periods when they are contracted out. Contracting out means that a person has opted to join an occupational scheme or a personal pensions scheme or stakeholder pension. While contacted out, a person will pay lower National Insurance Contributions on part of earnings or some of the contributions paid by an employee and employer are 'rebated' and paid into the occupational pension scheme or other pension scheme. This is discussed more fully further on in this book.

Increasing your state pension

There are a number of ways in which you can increase your State Pension, particularly if you have been presented with a pension forecast which shows lack of contributions and a diminished state pension. You can fill gaps in your pension contributions or you can defer your state pension. HM Revenue and Customs have a help line on 0845 915 5996 to check your record and to receive advice on whether you have gaps and how to fill them.

Filling gaps in your record

For people reaching State Pension Age on, or after, 6th April 2010, you need only 30 qualifying years for the full pension. Depending on your pension age your working life may be from 44 to 52 years. Therefore, under the post April 2010 rules, you can have substantial gaps in your record without any reduction in your basic pension.

If you wish to plus gaps in your contributions, normally you can go back 6 years to fill gaps in your record. However, if you will reach State Pension Age before April 5th 2015, special rules let you fill any gaps up to six years in total going back as far as 6th April 1975. You can make class 3 contributions to fill the gap, each contribution costs £12.05 so a full years worth costs 52 times 12.05 = £626.60. Making class three contributions can't increase your additional state pension. However Class 3 contributions do count towards the state bereavement benefits that your wife, husband or civil partner could claim if you were to die.

Deferring your state pension

Another way to boost your state pension is to delay its commencement. You can put off drawing your pension for as long as you like, there is no time limit. You must defer your whole pension, including any additional or graduated pensions and you earn an addition to the lump sum or a bigger cash sum.

In the past, if you put off drawing your own pension and your wife was getting a pension based on your NI record, her pension would also have to be deferred and she would have to agree to this. From 6th April 2010 onwards, husbands and civil partners as well as wives may be able to claim a pension based on their partners record. But a change to the rules now means that, if you defer your pension and your wife, husband or civil partner claims on your record, they no longer have to defer their pension as well.

If your pension has already started to be paid, you can decide to stop payments in order to earn extra pension or lump sum. But you can only defer your pension once. You can earn an increase in the pension when it does start of 1% for every five weeks you put off the pension. This is equivalent to an increase of 10.4% for each whole year.

Alternatively, if you put off claiming your pension for at least a whole year, you can earn a one-off lump sum instead of extra pension. The lump sum is taxable but only at the top rate you were paying before getting the lump sum. Whatever the size of the sum it does not mean that you move tax brackets.

The Pension Service publishes a detailed guide to deferring your Statepension.

Seewww.direct.gov.uk/prod consum dg/groups/dg digitalassets/
@dg/@en/@over50/documents/digitalasset/dg 180189.pdf

Carers allowance

This is a benefit for people who care for someone who is in
receipt of either Attendance Allowance or the Disability Living
Allowance care component at either the middle or higher rate.
You would be eligible for this allowance if you regularly spend 35
hours a week or more caring for someone. You do not have to be
related to or living to that person. Carers allowance is not
affected by any savings or income that you have, except any
earnings or benefits paid to replace earnings. It is not dependant
on NI contributions and it is taxable. If you are entitled to carers
allowance you will normally get a NI contribution credited to
your record. To get carerss allowance you must:

- Be aged 16 or over at the time of your claim
- Be living in the UK
- Not be in full time education (over 21 hours per week)
- Not earn more than £100 per week, once allowable
  expenses are deducted.

Carers allowance	Weekly rate
Basic allowance	£55.55 (2011-2012)

Top-up benefits

These types of benefits can be claimed to top up income if you
do not have enough to live on. Which benefit you can claim very
much depends on your circumstances.

Income Support

This is a benefit to cover essential living expenses. It is a means-tested benefit. To qualify, you don't need to have paid National insurance Contributions and it isn't taxable. You may qualify for Income Support if the following apply:

- Your capital is £16,000 or less (this means savings, pension, property and so on)
- Your weekly income is low
- You are aged 16 or over and under the age you can receive pension credit
- Neither you or your partner works full time. This means for you 16 hours or more or for a partner 21 hours or more.
- You are 'habitually resident' or have a 'right to reside' in the UK
- You are in a group that is eligible to claim income support. This includes people who are entitled to carer's allowance and lone parents with very young children.

Income Support can be claimed by calling the jobcentre Plus claim line on 0800 055 6688.

Income Support Rates

Single person under 25	£53.45
Single person over 45	£67.50
Lone parent under 18	£53.45
Lone parent 18 or over	£67.50
Couple both under 18	£53.45

Couple both under 18 higher rate	£80.75
Couple one under 18, one under 25	£53.45
Couple one under 18, one 25 and over	£67.50
Couple both 18 or over	£105.95
Dependent children	£62.33
Premiums-family, lone parent	£17.40

Further premiums

There are a range of further Income Support premiums payable. Further information can be obtained from the Department of Work and pensions.

Pension Credit
This is a means-tested benefit for people who have reached the qualifying age, which is 65 for men and 60 for women, but bear in mind that this is being steadily increased. To make a claim call the Pension Credit Application line 0800 99 1234.

Pension Credit Rates for 2011-2012
Standard minimum guarantee   **Weekly rates**

Single	£137.35
Couple	£209.70
Additional amount for severe disability-couple one qualifies	£55.30
Couple-both qualify	£110.60
Additional amount for carers	£31

Housing Benefit

Housing benefit is a benefit for people on low income to help them pay their rent. You may be able to get housing benefit if you are on other benefits or work part time or full time on a low income.

To get housing benefit in the first place you must pay rent. It doesn't matter who the landlord is, whether private or public sector. You can also claim housing benefit if you rent a room in a hostel or are a boarder. You can claim it if you share a house or flat as point or sub-tenants. You cannot get housing benefit if you rent your home from the Crown, or you are 16 or 17 or have been in care.

Only one member of a couple who live together can claim housing benefit. You must also live in the accommodation for which you are claiming benefit.

Students may be able to claim housing benefit, but special rules will apply.

UK Resident

You must be living in the UK to claim housing benefit. If you are from overseas or have recently arrived in the UK you may have difficulty claiming housing benefit.

Income and capital

To get housing benefit you must have income and capital below a certain level. Capital means savings, land, property or anything else that could provide you with an income. If you have more than £16,000 in capital you will not get housing benefit, unless you are getting the guarantee part of pension credit. If you have capital of over £6,000 you will be assumed to have some income from that capital.

If you are getting income support or income based jobseekers allowance, you will automatically be within the income and capital limits for housing benefits. If you are in pension credit and get the guarantee credit (whether on its own or with the savings credit) you will also automatically get the maximum housing benefit amount.

How much benefit can you get?

How much benefit you will get depends on how much rent you pay, what income you have and where you live. The rules for HB allowance are changing which are outlined below. If you pay rent to a private landlord, the rent your housing benefit will cover will normally be restricted to an amount set by the rent officer. When you make a new claim for housing benefit your local authority will normally calculate how much rent your housing benefit can cover suing the Local Authority Housing Allowance Rules. In some cases, it is possible for your housing benefit entitlement to be more than your rent, by up to £15 (see below for rule changes after April 2011). In many cases, however, the amount of HB that you are entitled to will not cover the full amount and you will have to make up the shortfall. There are different rules concerning applications for HB before and after 7th April 2008 and these rules can be obtained from the local authority.

Changes to housing benefit after April 2011

If you are making a new claim for housing benefit these changes will affect you after April 2011. If you are already claiming housing benefit, these changes are likely to affect the amount that you get towards your rent. The changes are a result of a root and branch overall of the benefit system, in the light of perceived changes needed as a result of the escalating bill.

From 1ˢᵗ April 2011, the rates for Local Housing Allowance will be reduced across the country. The maximum weekly excess of £15 will be removed. There will be a limit on payments so that the Local Housing Allowance does not exceed:

- £250 per week for a one bedroom property (including shared accommodation)
- £290 a week for a two bedroom property
- £340 a week for a three bedroom property
- £400 a week for a four bedroom property

The maximum rate of HB will be limited to a four-bedroom property. There will be help for disabled people towards the cost of an extra bedroom if they need an overnight carer.

Shared room rate

This currently applies to single people under the age of 25 living in accommodation that they rent from a private landlord. This will be extended to people under 35. This means that people under 35 will no longer receive HB based on one bedroom self-contained accommodation.

The above outline of housing benefit is very brief. The local authority in your area will be able to furnish you with full details.

Council tax and the tenant

Council tax is based on properties, or dwellings, and not individual people.

This means that there is one bill for each individual dwelling, rather than separate bills for each person. The number and type of people who live in the dwelling may affect the size of the final bill. A discount of 25% is given for people who live alone. Each property is placed in a valuation band with different properties paying more or less depending on their individual value. Tenants who feel that their home has been placed in the wrong valuation band can appeal to their local authority council tax department.

Who has to pay the council tax?

In most cases the tenant occupying the dwelling will have to pay the council tax. However, a landlord will be responsible for paying the council tax where there are several households living in one dwelling. This will usually be hostels, bedsits and other non-self contained flats where people share things such as cooking and washing facilities. The council tax on this type of property remains the responsibility of the landlord even if all but one of the tenants move out. Although the landlord has the responsibility for paying the council tax, he/she will normally try to pass on the increased cost through rents. However, as we have seen, there is a set procedure for a landlord to follow if he/she wishes to increase rent.

Council tax benefits available for those on low income

Tenants on very low income, except for students, will usually be able to claim council tax benefit. This can cover up to 100% of the council tax.

Tenants with disabilities may be entitled to further discounts. Tenants who are not responsible for individual council tax, but pay it through their rent, can claim housing benefit to cover the increase.

The rules covering council tax liability can be obtained from a Citizens Advice Bureau or from your local authority council tax department.

Working tax credit

Working Tax Credit is a payment to top up the earnings of working people on low incomes, whether they are employed or self-employed. You may be entitled to Working Tax Credit if you:

- Are in paid work, and
- Expect to work for at least four weeks, and
- Are aged 16 or over, responsible for at least one child and work at least 16 hours a week, or
- Are over 16 and have a disability (including Parkinson's) which puts you at a disadvantage in getting a job, are receiving some form of disability benefit and work at least 16 hours a week, or
- Are aged 25 or over and work at least 30 hours in a week, or

- Are aged 50 or over, are returning to work after time spent on qualifying out-of-work benefits and work at least 16 hours a week.

Working Tax Credit is comprised of a number of elements, including:

- Couples
- Lone parents
- Those working 30 hours or over
- Disabled workers
- People aged over 50 or over returning to work after a period of benefits.

The full range of Working Tax Credits available can be obtained from www.hmrc.gov.uk

Job Seekers Allowance (JSA)

This is the main form of benefit for people of working age who are out of work or work less than 16 hours per week. If you are eligible this benefit will be paid while you are looking for work. To get jobseekers allowance you must be available for, capable of and actively seeking work, aged 18 or over but below State Pension Age. JSA isn't usually paid to those under 18 except in special cases.

There are two types of jobseekers allowance, contribution based and income based Jobseekers Allowance. Contribution based JSA is based on NI contributions, whilst income based is based on savings and income. You may get this if you have not paid enough NIC's and you are on a low income.

Jobseekers Allowance Payments

Contribution based JSA	Amount
Aged 16-24	£53.45
Aged 25 and over	£67.50

Income based JSA	Amount
Single person under 25	£53.45
Single person 25 or over	£67.50
Couples and civil partners (aged 18 or over)	£105.95
Lone parent (under 18)	£53.45
Lone parent (over 18)	£67.50

This benefit can be claimed by calling Jobcentre plus on 0800 055 6688.

Other benefits available

There are a few other types of benefits available, such as National Insurance credits for parents and carers. These types of credits are aimed at protecting basic state pension rights and bereavement benefit rights when you are not paying NI because you are looking after someone. Your local Jobcentre Plus office can supply you with more information.

The Social Fund

The Social Fund consists of several grants and loans you can apply for if you have a low income. You can get grants for the following, subject to eligibility:

- Funeral payments

- Maternity needs
- Extra income during periods of very cold weather
- Items that you might need to help you stay in the community.

In addition to the Social Fund you may be able to get a budgeting loan or a crisis loan. For further details of Social fund and other payments contact your local Jobcentre Plus.

Winter Fuel payments

Winter-fuel payment is an annual tax-free payment for people who have reached pension credit qualifying age. It is not affected by your savings or assets and won't affect any other benefit that you receive.

To claim, contact the Winter Fuel Payments Helpline, on 0845 915 1515.

You can also get free health benefits if you are on a low income and get Income Support related ESA, Income Support or income based Job Seekers Allowance. These benefits include free prescriptions, eye tests, free dental treatment, glasses and expenses to and from hospital. To claim health benefits on the low-income scheme, you will need to complete form HC1, available from your Jobcentre Plus or by calling 0845 850 1166.

The next chapter deals with general advice for the person living with Parkinson's disease which will prove invaluable for the future. Some of this has already been covered generally throughout this book but is now covered in more depth.

****

Chapter 10

Living and Coping with Parkinson's Disease- General Advice

When a person first receives a diagnosis of Parkinson's disease, it can be very stressful and also confusing, both for the individual and family and friends. It is crucial, at the outset, that advice and information is available.

One of the most important factors in the life of someone with Parkinson's disease, particularly someone who has been newly diagnosed, is that of ongoing support. There is a lot of support out there, not least the umbrella groups such as Parkinson's UK who can be contacted on 0808 800 0303 e mail hello@parkinsons.org.uk or online at www. parkinsons.org.uk.

In addition, there are Parkinson's disease nurse specialists who are community based or based in a hospital. Their numbers have expanded over the years although there is not yet one in every area. They are registered nurses who have specialised in the area of Parkinson's disease and they have broad experience in neurology or the care of elderly people. Their work involves assessing individual care needs, enhancing and promoting quality of life and preventing, or at least minimising the complications associated with Parkinson's disease. Typical complications can include problems with mobility, urinary problems, depression, and the side effects of medication.

Therapies for Parkinson's disease

Parkinson's disease can interfere, to a greater or lesser extent, with many day-to-day activities. The aim of therapies is to ease these difficulties by helping you to learn the knowledge and skills that you will need to continue with a normal life. There are three main therapies available, physiotherapy, occupational therapy and speech and language therapy.

Physiotherapy

A physiotherapist will assess your needs by looking at the difficulties that you have with movement and general mobility. The aim of the physiotherapist is to help you achieve the greatest level of activity possible. They will teach you how to manage the physical problems associated with Parkinson's disease.

Beware of those who call themselves physiotherapists. A Qualified physiotherapist will be a member of the Chartered Society of Physiotherapists. Each person will specialise in a different area of physiotherapy, as with most other professions and not all physiotherapists have the required expertise in neurological disorders. Physiotherapists interested in neurological disorders will be senior practitioners and will often be termed neurophysiotherapists.

Physiotherapy will help you move more normally and with less effort. Physiotherapy is not about routine exercise, as has already been outlined in this book, but about learning skills and techniques to assist you with coping with problems that arise with the onset and development of the disease. Certain basic tasks, which you have found easy all your life, such as tying a tie or doing up your shoelaces can become a chore when you have Parkinson's. Physiotherapy will teach you certain techniques and provide learning strategies, such as talking through a task while doing it or relying on visual targets to improve performance. These approaches are known as cueing.

Stiffness and poor posture also comes with Parkinson's. Muscles and joints will stiffen up over time making it increasingly harder to walk and relax. Physiotherapists can help to relieve this muscle and joint stiffness. Physiotherapists can also advise you about appropriate exercises that will help you, such as swimming or the Alexander technique.

Occupational therapy

Occupational therapists will assist you in those daily aspects of life that have become increasingly more difficult, such as looking after yourself and others, and also with work and leisure. It can also be difficult for you to travel where you want, because of mobility problems. Occupational therapists will work with you to improve your life by identifying areas of particular difficulty and devising a programme specifically for you to help you overcome these problems. A qualified occupational therapist will be state registered and have a degree (BSc (Hons) OT) or diploma (DipCot). As with physiotherapists occupational therapists specialise in different areas. These occupational therapists who have specialised in neurological disorders might be members of NANOT (National Association of Neurological OT's) or have done some further specialised training after initially qualifying as an occupational therapist.

Speech and language therapists

A speech and language therapist will work with Parkinson's sufferers and also, where necessary, with family or carers. They will identify where the difficulties impact on lifestyle, such as using the telephone or when conversing in shops or at work. Therapy will include exercises that work on improving voice loudness and intelligibility of speech generally. Communication can be affected by the types of swallowing difficulties encountered by people with Parkinson's, which include difficulties controlling saliva, difficulty chewing harder foods and problems with swallowing generally. Some may experience coughing or choking episodes while eating. A speech and language therapist will assess swallowing problems and provide advice on the easiest food and drinks and also the safest approach to eating and drinking. It is highly advisable to see a therapist as soon as possible after your initial diagnosis of Parkinson's. Your family doctor or consultant will usually make the referral to see a therapist

Driving and Parkinson's

A diagnosis of Parkinson's does not always mean that you will have to cease driving. However, you must by law inform the Driver and Vehicle Licensing Agency (DVLA). You can continue to drive after informing the DVLA until they inform you other wise. If you or your family or friends have any concerns, however, you should stop driving and discuss the matter with your doctor.

The DVLA assesses each case individually and may issue either a restricted licence, (restricted to a number of years or to a vehicle with adaptations) or an unrestricted licence. Both of these will allow you to continue driving once you have been diagnosed with Parkinson's. However, the DVLA can also decide that you should not be allowed to drive for a specified period. If you are not happy with the DVLA's decision then you can appeal asking them to reconsider or you can appeal in a magistrate's court.

When you contact the DVLA, you will need to complete two forms, PK1 'Medical in confidence' available from the DirectGov website and a shorter medical questionnaire detailing your symptoms and you may be required to undergo further medical assessment and possibly retake the practical part of the driving test. Medicals and driving tests are free to those newly diagnosed with Parkinson's. A more detailed booklet is available from www.parkinsons.org.uk.

Parkinson's medication and driving

The side effects that some people might experience from their medication can affect driving. Dopamine agonists can cause drowsiness, sometime severe. You need to be aware of this and consult the literature about side effects provided with your medication. You can also get advice from your doctor.

Mobility centres and driving assessment.

Mobility centres provide information and advice on driving for any person who is disabled and uses a car, either as a driver or a passenger. They will also offer assessments on your ability to drive a vehicle. There are a number of mobility centres in the UK, again information can be obtained from the DVLA website or from www. parkinsons.org.uk.

Priority parking and the Blue Badge Scheme

You may qualify for parking concessions through the Blue Badge Scheme if you have a severe disability and also qualify for the higher rate of the mobility component of the Disability Living Allowance (see chapter on benefits). The Blue Badge Scheme enables people who have certain disabilities to park closer to shops and the services that they need to get to. The badge applies whether they are driver or passenger in a vehicle. More information can be obtained from the DirectGov website www.directgov.co.uk.

In addition to the above, if you are disabled and qualify for DLA or the War Pensioners Mobility Supplement you may also be eligible for a car tax exemption.

Car insurance and Parkinson's

If you have been diagnosed with Parkinson's you should inform your car insurance company as any changes in your health may affect your ability to drive and render your policy invalid. It is also an offence under the Road Traffic Act not to inform your insurer of changes of circumstances. You must also inform your insurers about any adaptations to your vehicle. Insurers will want to know about any disabilities or health problems, particularly if there have been any restrictions imposed on your licence. Insurers are not allowed to refuse insurance to disabled drivers unless they can justify it. Any insurance premium has to be based on a reasonable assessment of risk. If you feel that an insurer has behaved unreasonably or has not acted within the remit of the Equality Act 2010 (see Parkinson's and employment) you should complain directly to the insurer. If the response of the Insurer is not satisfactory then you should go to the Financial Services Ombudsman (address at the back of the book).

Adaptations to vehicles for drivers with Parkinson's

If you have Parkinson's and it is impacting on your driving comfort and safety, then you can get your vehicle adapted to suit your particular condition. There are motoring accessories available for people with upper or lower body disabilities or both, which include:

- Hand controls to operate the accelerator or break
- Aids to help you turn the steering wheel with greater ease
- Accessories to help you get in and out of your vehicle such as cushions, covers and support
- Adapted mirrors for greater vision
- Different types of seat belts and harnesses
- Lifts and wheelchair hoists.

This list is not exclusive there are a number of adaptations which would be recommended at the time of fitting.

Dropped kerbs

A dropped kerb can make it easier to access your vehicle. For this you would normally apply to your local county council (or your local authority who can advise). More information is available on the DirectGov website.

Employment and Parkinson's

When you are diagnosed with Parkinson's this will, if you are in employment, cause anxiety as to your future, particularly as the condition progresses. Because Parkinson's differs with each person, you may or may not have to change the way you work or change employment. You may, however, feel that you would benefit from some changes in your work environment and you shouldn't be afraid to raise this with your employer.

The Equality Act 2010

This Act drew together all the strands of previous legislation, such as the Sex Discrimination Act, Disability Discrimination Act and Equal pay legislation. The Act will directly affect people whose condition is affected by Parkinson's. Basically, the Act stipulates that an employer shall not discriminate, directly or indirectly, against a person with disabilities. Very importantly, it also states that an employer should make reasonable adjustments to accommodate disabled people, which could include:

- The provision of equipment
- Changes in work practices
- Changes in work hours, such as flexible or reduced hours
- Allowing extra rest time.

If you are a member of a trade union then advice can be sought from representatives. In addition, information about employment issues is available from the Equality and Human Rights Commission (England, Wales and Scotland) or Equality Commission for Northern Ireland.

Chapter 11

People who care for Parkinson's Sufferer's

Definition of a carer

We have all heard of the word "carer". This denotes a number of things. A carer can be someone who looks after their mother or father or looks after someone else in the family or a friend in an unpaid capacity. A carer is quite different to a home help.

Someone who is in the position of a carer for a person who has been diagnosed with Parkinson's can claim benefits in certain circumstances, access help and support from social services and also receive priority support from local health services. Carer's benefits are outlined in the chapter on welfare benefits.

Providing care to a person with Parkinson's

As the symptoms associated with Parkinson's will change over time, the nature of the care that is provided will also, of necessity, change with that person's needs. For example, in the early stages of Parkinson's the level of care needed may be minimal. It is at this early stage that it is important to gather as much information as you possibly can about the condition so you can become acquainted with the possible future needs of the person. You can gather information from a number of sources, the Internet, for example from Parkinson's UK www.parkinsons.org.uk or from medical and social services providers.

Many people with Parkinson's stay independent for years after their initial diagnosis and won't really need a lot of care. It is important during this time to display a positive attitude which can be of great benefit to your partner or relative/friend and can make a significant difference to how they cope with Parkinson's. There are a number of ways that you as a carer can assist, such as encouraging them to lead as active and normal a life as is possible under the circumstances and allowing them to do as much for themselves as possible.

If you feel that you need further training and advice in this area there are a number of courses, and informal groupings, available for carer's which explore the issues involved and allow you to meet other people in the same circumstances. There are useful contacts listed at the end of this chapter and at the back of the book.

Talking to health professionals

Your GP will be the first person you should talk to about your caring responsibilities. Carer's are given special consideration because of their role and the pressure that comes with that role. It always helps to compile a list of your needs and of the concerns that you wish to discuss with your doctor. Again, Parkinson's UK has useful information relating to discussing things with your doctor.

Following discussions with your GP, he/she will then, through the primary care team provide support and advice and:

- Arrange home visits to you or the person that you care for
- Arrange appointments for you and the person that you care for at the same time
- Supply repeat prescriptions to be delivered to your local pharmacy
- Put you in touch with other sources of support and advice such as other voluntary advice agencies
- Provide any letters of support that may be required for benefit departments or other agencies, such as the Blue Badge Scheme.

The Carer's Register

A carer's register is a database compiled by (some) surgeries that will enable staff to identify carer's and also those in receipt of care. The register is used to help get the right services at the right time, provide clear information about other relevant services and receive up-to-date information about events for carer's. In addition, the register will ensure that appointments are offered at appropriate times and that outpatient appointments and letters make clear that the person is a carer.

Time off from caring

Time of from caring is known as a 'Respite Break'. Time off from caring responsibilities is very important. Taking a break can help alleviate the anxieties and depression that accompany the role of carer. Respite breaks don't always mean that you have to go away somewhere, they can be given in a variety of ways, such as a social services care worker taking over for a while, or someone from a charity such as Crossroads Care (address at the back of the book) coming to the home regularly to care for the person with

Parkinson's. In addition, the person that you care for can spend some time at a day centre or can spend short periods in a care home. All of this will depend on the circumstances at the time.

Carer's assessments

The local authority in your area has responsibility for arranging services that can help you take a break from caring. This will be achieved through a carer's assessment. Social services then use the assessment to decide what services to provide. You would normally initiate the assessment by visiting the social services department of the local council and asking for an assessment for the person that you care for and also for yourself as the carer.

The social services department will also carry out a financial assessment, which may mean that either you or the person being cared for will be responsible for all or some of the services provided. The decision to charge will be according to means.

Carers and employment rights

If you are in the position where you are caring for someone with Parkinson's and also working at the same time, you may find that the pressure on you as a person increases significantly. Carer's have statutory rights at work that can help reduce this pressure and also help to meet other needs. Employers also may be able to offer additional flexibility through their own policies and procedures.

Telling your employer about your role as a carer
There is no legal obligation to inform your employer about your role as carer. If you decide to tell your employer then make sure

that you are fully aware of your statutory rights. You can find detailed information about your rights and employer's responsibilities from Carers UK   www.carersuk.org and DirectGov.

Statutory rights for carer's

The main law protecting carer's in the workplace is the Work and Families Act 2006 and the Employment Rights Act 1996, which give working carer's rights to help them manage work and caring. This includes the right to request flexible work and leave entitlement. In Northern Ireland they are called the Work and Families (Northern Ireland) Order 2006 and the Employment Rights (Northern Ireland) Order 2006. Your employment status can affect your entitlement to statutory rights. If you are self-employed, on a short term contract or employed through an agency you may not be covered by these rights. If this applies to you, contact ACAS on 08457 47 47 47 for further advice.

Your employer may already have procedures in place to support carer's. This will usually be within the staff handbook or the intranet. The size and nature of the employer will determine whether or not they have publicized these rights. The public sector or large private sector employers are usually better at doing this.

As a working carer, you are likely to need a range of support, from access to a telephone to leave arrangements that work around the hospital visits etc of the person with Parkinson's.

You have a right to a ' reasonable' amount of time off work to deal with an emergency involving a dependant, such as a disruption or breakdown in care arrangements, a dependant falling ill or time to make better long term arrangements for a dependant. The right also includes some protection from victimisation or dismissal when you take time off. It is at the employer's discretion whether the leave is paid or unpaid.

Useful websites for carers to gain further information about the role of a carer and rights and responsibilities

Carers Direct www.nhs/carersdirect

Carers direct gives information and advice to carers

Care Directions www.caredirections.co.uk

Care Directions gives advice and information on health and care issues for older people

Carers Federation www.carersfederation.co.uk

The Carers Federation provides support for carers and for others with medical and mental health issues.

Carers UK www.carersuk.org

Carers UK is the main voice of carers in the UK providing advice and information and also campaigning on behalf of carers.

Crossroads care www.crossroads.org.uk

Crossroads provides support for carers and those being cared for.

Disabled Living Foundation www.dlf.org.uk
The Disabled Living foundation is a charity that provides advice about disability aids.

Employers for carers www.employersforcarers.org
Employers for carers provides practical advice for employers concerning the support of carers in their workforce.

Relate www.relate.org.uk
Relate provides relationship counselling and support services.

Relatives and residents association www.relres.org
The Relatives and Residents association provides advice and information on care homes and support for those with emotional concerns.

The Outsiders www.outsiders.org.ukThe Outsiders is a social and peer support network of disabled people, offering advice for people who have concerns about sexual or personal relationships.

The Princess Royal Trust for Carers www.carers.org
The Princess royal trust offers information and support for carers.

Young Carers Initiative www.youngcarer.com
The Young Carers Initiative offers advice and support to young carers and their families.

Useful Addresses

Ability Net Central England
PO Box 94
Warwick
Warwickshire.
CV34 5WS
Freephone: 0800 269545
Web: www.abilitynet.org.uk
Information on specialist assistive
Technology to help people with
Any disability to use a computer.

Age Concern England
Astral house
1268 London Road
London
SW16 4ER
Tel: 020 8765 7200
Helpline: 0800 009966
www.ageconcern.org.uk
Researches into the needs of elderly
People and is involved in policy-making.

Benefits Enquiry Line
Tel: 0800 882200
Minicom: 0800 243355
www.dwp.gov.uk
N. Ireland 0800 220674

Warbreck House
Warbreck Hill Road

Blackpool
FY2 0YE
Email: bel-customer-services@dwp.gsi.gov.uk

Government agency giving information and
Advice on sickness and disability benefits for
People with disabilities and their carers.

British Association / College of
Occupational Therapists
106-114 Borough High Street
London
SE1 1LB
Tel:020 7357 6480 or
020 7450 2330
www.cot.org.uk

Information about all aspects of Occupational
Therapy. An S.A.E. requested.

Carers UK
20 Great Dover Street
London
SE1 4LX
Tel: 020 7378 4 999
Carers' line: 0808 808 7777
www.carersuk.org

Offers information and support to all people
Who are unpaid carers, looking after others
With medical or other problems.

Chartered Society of Physiotherapy
14 Bedford Row
London
WC1R 4ED
Tel:020 7306 6666
www.csp.org.uk

Information about all aspects of physiotherapy.

Citizens Advice Bureaux
(National Association of CABs)
Myddelton House
115-123 Pentonville Road
London
N1 9LZ
www.citizensadvice.org.uk

HQ of national charity offering a wide variety of
Practical and legal advice. Network of local
Branches throughout the UK listed in phone
Books and Yellow Pages under Counselling and Advice.

Counsel and Care
Twyman House
Bonny Street
London
NW1 9PG
Tel: 020 7241 8555
Helpline: 0845 300 7585
(Mon-Fri 10am-4pm except Wed 10am-1pm)
www.counselandcare.org.uk

Information and advice on homes,community
Care and housing with care.

Crossroads Caring for Carers
10 Regent Place
Rugby
Warwickshire
CV21 2PN
Helpline: 0845 450 0350
www.crossroads.org.uk

Supports and delivers high-quality service for
Carers and people with care needs via its local branches.

Dial UK
St Catherine's
Tickhill Road
Doncaster
S. Yorkshire
DN4 8QN
Tel / texphone: 01302 310123
www.dialuk.info

Nationwide network offering information and
Advice on all aspects of disability ; 130 drop -in
Centres run by and for people with disabilities.
Disabled Living Foundation
380-384 Harrow Road
London
W9 2HU
Tel: 020 7289 6111
www.dlf.org.uk

Provides information to disabled and elderly people
On all kinds of equipment in order to promote
Their independence and quality of life.

DVLA
Driver and Vehicle Licensing Agency
Swansea
SA6 7JL
Tel: 0870 600 0301
www.dvla.gov.uk

Provides information about
Medical conditions, driving licences, learning
To drive, entitlement to drive

European Parkinson's Disease Association
(EPDA)
4 Golding Road
Sevenoaks
Kent
TN13 3NJ
Tel: 01732 457683
www.epda.eu.com

Umbrella body for network of international
Parkinson's disease groups, campaigning on behalf
Of all suffers. Information leaflets on request.
An S.A.E. requested.

Homecraft Rolyan
Nunn Brook Road
Huthwaite

Sutton in Ashfield
Notts
NG17 2HU
Tel: 0844 412 4330
 (For International Visitors
Tel: +44 1623 448706)
www.homecraft-rolyan.com

Mail order company offering a wide range
Of items and equipment suitable for people with disabilities.

Institute for Complementary and
Natural Medicine
Can- Mezzanine
32-36 Loman Street
London
SE1 0EH
Tel: 08454 456 2537
www.i-c-m.org.uk

Umbrella group for complementary medicine
Organisation. Offers information, safe choice to
Public.

Keep Able
3-4 Sterling Park
Pedmore Road
Brierley Hill
W. Midlands
DY51 1TB
Tel: 0870 520 2122 or
Tel: 084 4888 1338

Fax: 013 8448 0260
www.keepable.co.uk

Nationwide chain of stores, advising
And suppling a wide range of products
For people with disabilities.

Leonard Cheshire
66 South Lambeth Road
London
SW8 1RL
Tel: 020 3242 0200
www.lcdisability.org
Email: info@lcdisability.org

Offers care, support and a wide range of
Information for disabled people aged between
18 and 65 years in the UK and worldwide to
encourage independent living. Has respite
and residential homes; offers holidays
and rehabilitation.

Mobilise
National HQ
Ashwellthorpe
Norwich
NR16 1EX
Tel: 01508 489449
www.mobilise.info

Provides information for drivers with
A disability on a wide range of issues.

Motability
Motability Operations
City Gate House
22 Southwark Bridge Road
London
SE1 9HB
Tel:0845 456 4566
www.motability.co.uk

Helps driver with disabilities to access specialist
Cars and funding with Motability car schemes.

National Institute for Health and Clinical
Excellence (NICE)
MidCity Place
71 High Holborn
London
WC1V 6NA
Tel: 0845 003 7780
www.nice.org.uk

Provides national guidance on the
Promotion of good health and treatment
of ill-health. Patient information leaflets
Are available for each piece of guidance issued.

NHS Direct
Tel: 0845 4647 (24 hours, 365days a year)
www.nhsdirect.nhs.uk

Parkinson's UK
National Office

215 Vauxhall Bridge Road
London
Hepline: 0808 800 0303
Tel: 020 7931 8080
Fax: 020 7233 9908
www.parkinsons.org.uk

Offers information and support via its local groups
Has nurse specialists and welfare department,
And funds research into Parkinson's disease.

Patients' Association
PO Box 935
Harrow
Middlesex
HA1 3YJ
Helpline: 0845 608 4455
Tel: 020 8423 9111
www.patients-association.com
Email: helpline@patients-association.com

Provides advice on patients' rights, leaflets and
A directory of self-help groups.

RADAR: The Disability Network
12 City Forum
250 City Road
London
EC1V 8AF
Tel: 020 7250 3222
Minicom: 020 7250 4119
www.radar.org.uk Email: radar@radar.org.uk

Campaigns to improve the rights and care of
Disabled people. Sells special key to access locked disabled toilets.

Royal College of Speech and Language
Therapy
2 White Hart Yard
London
SE1 1NX
Tel: 020 7378 1200
www.rcslt.org

Information about all aspects of speech
And language therapy.

Tourism for All
C/O Vitalise
Shap Road Industrial Estate
Shap Road
Kendal
Cumbria
LA9 6NZ
Tel: 0845 124 9974
www.tourismforall.org.uk

Provides information to people with disabilities
On transport, holiday accommodation,
Activity holidays are respite care establishments
In the UK and abroad .
See Vitalise below.

Vitalise (previously Winged Fellowship Trust)
12 City Forum

250 City Road
London
EC1V 8AF
Tel: 0845 345 1972
Fax: 0845 345 1978
www.vitalise.org.uk

Offers holidays at their own centres and overseas
And respite care for people with severe disabilities by
Prviding voluntary carers. Also arrages holidays for
People with Alzheimer's disease/dementia and
Their carers.

YPN (Younger Parkinson's Network)
National helpline : 0808 800 0303
www.http://yap-web.net

The young-onset self-help group of the Parkinson's
Disase Society and is designed really for those of
Working age. There are around 1,300 members
Of YPN , many of them in their early 20s and 30s.
Has a magazine, local meetings and conference every
2 years.

Parkinson's UK Support Group
Townsend Hall
Shipston on Stour
Warks
CV36 4AE
Tel: 0844 225 3644
www.parkinson.org.uk

David Rayner Centre
120 Cambridge Road
Great Shelford
Cambridege
CB22 5JT
Helpline: 080 8800 0303
www.parkinsons.org.uk

Network of local groups bringing people
With Parkinson's and their families
Together for support and help.

Parkinson's Home Care
Helping Hand Homecare
Arrow House
8-9 Church Street
Alcester
Warwickshire
B49 5AJ
Free phone: 0808 180 9455
www.helpinghandscare.co.uk

Support Group for Asian People
2 Valley Gardens
West Bridgford
Nottingham
NG2 6HG
Email: mkraca@kaura.me-uk

Specific Information for drivers

Driving and Parkinson's
Association of British Insurers (ABI) www.abi.org.uk

The ABI will assist you with any complaints that you may have about insurers

Department for Transport www.dft.gov.uk

The DFT aims to ensure that provisions for all motorists are acceptable, accessible and affordable.

Disability Alliance www.disability alliance.org

The Disability Alliance provides advice on benefits and services for people with disabilities.

Disabled Living Foundation www.dlf.org.uk

As above provides advice and information.

DVLA (Driver and Vehicle Licensing Agency) www.dvla.gov.uk

The DVLA will provide advice and information on all aspects of driving.

Mobilise www.mobilise.info

Mobilise provides help and support to disabled drivers and passengers.

Motability www.motability.co.uk
Motability helps to keep disabled drivers on the road.

Appendix 1

Sample medication log

As mentioned earlier in the chapter on finding and dealing with doctors and specialists, it is very important to keep a log of the medications that you take and when you take them, plus also the types of symptoms that you are experiencing. The below is an example which might help you.

Medication

Date	Time	Type and dosage	Symptoms/moods	Next dose

24 Hour record of symptoms

Date_____

Time	Medication dosage	Symptoms/moods
6am		
8am		
10am		
12noon		
2pm		
4pm		
6pm		
8pm		
10pm		
12am		
2am		
4am		

The purpose of the logs on the previous page is to ensure that you have an accurate record of what exactly is happening to you in order that both your doctor and anyone who interacts with you on a professional level understands and knows what is going on. As stated, it is likely that your doctor will have an accurate record, as this is their job, but others who deal with you may not.

Index

Additional state pension, 86
Aerobic fitness, 64
Agency workers, 73
Amantadine, 34
Anger, 46, 47
Anticholinergic drugs, 33
Arthritis, 29
Attendance allowance, 71
Benign tremor, 28
Blue Badge Scheme, 106, 111
Car insurance, 106
Cardiovascular conditioning, 65
Carer's assessments, 112
Carer's Register, 111
Carers allowance, 90
Carers and employment rights, 112
Cell implants, 38
Civil Partnerships Act 2004, 78
Class 1 contributions, 80
Class 2 contributions, 81
Class 3 contributions, 82
Contracting out, 87
Controlling nausea, 60
Council tax, 96, 97
Dancing, 65
Deep Brain Stimulation, 37
Denial, 47
Depression, 29, 45, 47
Diagnosis of Parkinson's disease, 27
Diet, 53
Disability Living Allowance, 69, 70, 90, 106

Dopamine, 32, 33, 105
Dopamine agonists, 33
Driver and Vehicle Licensing Agency (DVLA, 104
Driving and Parkinson's, 104, 128
Dropped kerbs, 107
Electro-Convulsive therapy, 46
Employment and Support Allowance, 74, 75, 76, 77, 83
Employment Rights Act 1996, 113
Enzyme inhibitors, 32
Equality Act 2010, 106, 108
Essential tremor, 29
Exercise, 63
Financial Services Ombudsman, 107
Flexibility, 66
Foetal implants, 39
Funeral payments, 99
General practitioner, 41
Home Responsibilities Protection, 82
Housing Benefit, 93
Incapacity benefit, 76
Income tax, 77
Job Seekers Allowance (JSA), 98
Jogging, 64
Lesioning, 37, 38
Levodopa, 32
Madopar, 32
Medications, 31
Minerals, 61
Mobility centres, 105
Moncamine oxidase B, 32
Muscle weakness, 63
National Insurance, 87
National Insurance Credits, 82

Neurophysiotherapists., 102
NI contribution credits, 81
Occupational therapy, 103
Osteoporosis, 54
Pallidotomy, 38
Parkinson's symptoms, 28, 29, 38, 63
Parkinson's UK, 48, 59, 67, 101, 109, 110, 127
Pension Credit, 74, 92
Physiotherapy, 102, 118
Positron emission tomography (PET), 28
Puree diets, 58
Qualifying for state pension, 78
Respite Break, 111
Self-employed, 81, 87
SERPS, 86
Severe Disablement Allowance, 76
Sinemet, 32
Single photon emission tomography (SPECT), 28
Social Fund, 99, 100
Speech and language therapists, 59, 104
State Earnings Related Pension, 86
State Pension, 77, 84, 85, 88, 98
State pensions for people over 80, 86
Statutory rights for carer's, 113
Statutory Sick pay, 72
Stem cells, 39
Stroke, 30
Support groups, 47
Surgery for Parkinson's Disease, 37
Swimming, 64
Thalamotomy, 38
The brain, 30
Therapies, 102

Underweight, 55
Vitamins, 61
War Pensioners Mobility Supplement, 106
Winter Fuel payments, 100
Work and Families Act 2006, 113
Working tax credit, 97

Emerald Publishing
www.emeraldpublishing.co.uk

20 Newton Road
Brighton BN7 2SH

Other titles in the Emerald Series:

Law
Guide to Bankruptcy
Conducting Your Own Court case
Guide to Consumer law
Creating a Will
Guide to Family Law
Guide to Employment Law
Guide to European Union Law
Guide to Health and Safety Law
Guide to Criminal Law
Guide to Landlord and Tenant Law
Guide to the English Legal System
Guide to Housing Law
Guide to Marriage and Divorce
Guide to The Civil Partnerships Act
Guide to The Law of Contract
The Path to Justice
You and Your Legal Rights
The Debt Collecting Merry Go Round

Health
Guide to Combating Child Obesity
Asthma Begins at Home

The Ultimate Nutrition Guide for Cancer Sufferers and Their
Friends and Family
The Ultimate Nutrition Guide for Osteoporosis Sufferers
The Sea Medicine Chest
Natures Aspirin

Music
How to Survive and Succeed in the Music Industry

General
A Practical Guide to Obtaining probate
A Practical Guide to Residential Conveyancing
Writing The Perfect CV
Keeping Books and Accounts-A Small Business Guide
Business Start Up-A Guide for New Business
Finding Asperger Syndrome in the Family-A Book of Answers
Writing Your Autobiography
Being a professional Writer

For details of the above titles published by Emerald go to:

www.emeraldpublishing.co.uk